Occupational Therapy Practice Guidelines for

Mental Health Promotion, Prevention, and Intervention for Children and Youth

Susan Bazyk, PhD, OTR/L, FAOTA
Professor, Occupational Therapy Program
Cleveland State University
School of Health Sciences
Cleveland, OH

Marian Arbesman, PhD, OTR/L
President, ArbesIdeas, Inc.
Consultant, AOTA Evidence-Based Practice Project
Clinical Assistant Professor, Department of Rehabilitation Science
State University of New York at Buffalo
New York

D1270656

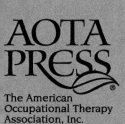

AOTA PRESS

The American
Occupational Therapy
Association, Inc.

AOTA Centennial Vision

We envision that occupational therapy is a powerful, widely recognized, science-driven, and evidence-based profession with a globally connected and diverse workforce meeting society's occupational needs.

AOTA Vision Statement

The American Occupational Therapy Association advances occupational therapy as the pre-eminent profession in promoting the health, productivity, and quality of life of individuals and society through the therapeutic application of occupation.

AOTA Mission Statement

The American Occupational Therapy Association advances the quality, availability, use, and support of occupational therapy through standard-setting, advocacy, education, and research on behalf of its members and the public.

AOTA Staff

Frederick P. Somers, *Executive Director*
Christopher M. Bluhm, *Chief Operating Officer*

Chris Davis, *Director, AOTA Press*
Ashley Hofmann, *Development/Production Editor*
Victoria Davis, *Digital/Production Editor*

Beth Ledford, *Director, Marketing*
Amanda Fogle, *Marketing Specialist*
Jennifer Folden, *Marketing Specialist*

The American Occupational Therapy Association, Inc.
4720 Montgomery Lane
Bethesda, MD 20814
301-652-AOTA (2682)
TDD: 800-377-8555
Fax: 301-652-7711
www.aota.org

To order: 1-877-404-AOTA (2682)

Disclaimers

This publication is designed to provide accurate and authoritative information in regard to the subject matter covered. It is sold or distributed with the understanding that the publisher is not engaged in rendering legal, accounting, or other professional service. If legal advice or other expert assistance is required, the services of a competent professional person should be sought.
—*From the Declaration of Principles jointly adopted by the American Bar Association and a Committee of Publishers and Associations*

It is the objective of the American Occupational Therapy Association to be a forum for free expression and interchange of ideas. The opinions expressed by the contributors to this work are their own and not necessarily those of the American Occupational Therapy Association.

ISBN-13: 978-1-56900-341-1
Library of Congress Control Number: 2013936086

Cover design by Jennifer Folden
Composition by Maryland Composition, Laurel, MD
Printing by Automated Graphics Systems, White Plains, MD

Contents

Figures, Boxes, and Tables

Acknowledgements

The series editor for this Practice Guideline is

Deborah Lieberman, MHSA, OTR/L, FAOTA
Director, Evidence-Based Practice
Staff Liaison to the Commission on Practice
American Occupational Therapy Association
Bethesda, MD

The authors acknowledge the following individuals for their contribution to the evidence-based literature review:

Susan Nochajski, PhD, OTR/L
Aarti Rego-Pereira, MS, OTR/L
Rachel Acquard Eising, MS, OTR/L
Jessica Williams Hoffarth, MS, OTR/L
Sara Zarinkelki, MS, OTR/L
Kelly Todd, MS, OTR/L
Diana Minardo, MS, OTR/L
Kyleen King, MS, OTR/L

The authors acknowledge and thank the following individuals for their participation in the content review and development of this publication:

Jan Hollenbeck, OTD, OTR/L
Leslie L. Jackson, MEd, OT/L, FAOTA
Tracy Jirikowic, PhD, OTR/L
Susan Nochajski, PhD, OTR/L
Sharon A. Ray, ScD, OTR/L
Deborah A. Whitcomb, MBA, MS, OTR/L
Tim Nanof, MSW
Sandy Schefkind, MS, OTR/L
Judy Thomas, MGA
Madalene Palmer

Note. The authors of this Practice Guideline have signed a Conflict of Interest statement indicating that they have no conflicts that would bear on this work.

Introduction

Purpose and Use of This Publication

> Raising children . . . is vastly more than fixing what is wrong with them. It is about identifying and nurturing their strongest qualities, what they own and are best at, and helping them find niches in which they can best live out these strengths. (Seligman & Csikszentmihalyi, 2000, p. 6)

Practice guidelines have been widely developed in response to the health care reform movement in the United States. Such guidelines can be a useful tool for improving the quality of health care, enhancing consumer satisfaction, promoting appropriate use of services, and reducing costs. The American Occupational Therapy Association (AOTA), which represents nearly 140,000 occupational therapists, occupational therapy assistants (see Appendix A), and students of occupational therapy, is committed to providing information to support decision making that promotes high-quality health care, wellness promotion, and educational services that are affordable and accessible to all.

Using an evidence-based perspective and key concepts from the second edition of the *Occupational Therapy Practice Framework: Domain and Process* (AOTA, 2008), this guideline provides an overview of the occupational therapy process for mental health promotion, prevention, and intervention for children and youth ages 3 to 21. This practice guideline is an update of one originally published in 2005 (Jackson & Arbesman, 2005) to incorporate evidence published since the first version. It defines the occupational therapy domain and process and interventions that occur within the boundaries of acceptable practice. This guideline does not discuss all possible methods of care, and although it does recommend some specific methods of care, the occupational therapist makes the ultimate judgment regarding the appropriateness of a given intervention in light of a specific person's circumstances, needs, and available evidence to support the intervention.

It is the intention of AOTA, through this publication, to help occupational therapists and occupational therapy assistants, as well as the individuals who manage, reimburse, or set policy regarding occupational therapy services, understand the contribution of occupational therapy in promoting mental health for children and youth ages 3 to 21. This guideline also can serve as a reference for teachers and other related services personnel, school principals and administrators, health care professionals, health care facility managers, education and health care regulators, third-party payers, and managed care organizations. Readers seeking evidence on occupational therapy for children ages 3 years or younger should refer to the *Occupational Therapy Practice Guidelines for Early Childhood: Birth Through 5 Years* (Frolek Clark & Kingsley, 2013).

This document may be used in any of the following ways:

- To assist occupational therapists and occupational therapy assistants in communicating about their services to external audiences
- To assist other health care providers, teachers, families and caregivers, mental health

providers, and program administrators in determining whether referral for occupational therapy services would be appropriate

- To assist third-party payers in determining the therapeutic need for occupational therapy
- To assist legislators, third-party payers, and administrators in understanding the professional education, training, and skills of occupational therapists and occupational therapy assistants
- To assist health and education planning teams in determining the developmental and educational need for occupational therapy
- To assist program developers, administrators, legislators, and third-party payers in understanding the scope of occupational therapy services
- To assist program evaluators and policy analysts in this practice area in determining outcome measures for analyzing the effectiveness of occupational therapy intervention
- To assist policy, education, and health care benefit analysts in understanding the appropriateness of occupational therapy services for mental health promotion in children and youth
- To assist occupational therapy educators in designing appropriate curricula that incorporate the role of occupational therapy for mental health promotion in children and youth.

The introduction to this guideline continues with a brief discussion of the domain and process of occupational therapy. This discussion is followed by a detailed description of the occupational therapy process for mental health promotion, including a summary of evidence from the literature regarding best practices with children and youth. Embedded within these descriptions are summaries of the results of a systematic review of evidence from the scientific literature regarding best practices in occupational therapy intervention for this population.

In addition, Appendix B contains a description of evidence-based practice as it relates to occupational therapy and the process used to conduct the evidence-based practice review related to children's mental health. All studies identified by the review, including those not specifically described in this section, are summarized in the evidence tables in Appendix C. Readers are encouraged to read the full articles for more details. Appendix D contains supplementary information about topics related to children's mental health, such as bullying and friendship issues, obesity, mental health literacy, sensory processing, structured leisure participation, and prevention of risky teen behaviors.

Domain and Process of Occupational Therapy

Occupational therapy practitioners'[1] expertise lies in their knowledge of occupation and of how engaging in occupations can be used to support health and participation in home, school, workplace, and community life (AOTA, 2008).

In 2008, the AOTA Representative Assembly adopted the second edition of the *Occupational Therapy Practice Framework: Domain and Process*. Informed by the first edition of the *Occupational Therapy Practice Framework* (AOTA, 2002), the previous *Uniform Terminology for Occupational Therapy* (AOTA, 1979, 1989, 1994), and the World Health Organization's *International Classification of Functioning, Disability and Health* (WHO, 2001), the *Framework* outlines the profession's domain and the process of service delivery within this domain.

Domain

A profession's *domain* articulates its sphere of knowledge, societal contribution, and intellectual or scientific activity. The occupational therapy profession's

---

[1]When the term *occupational therapy practitioner* is used in this document, it refers to both occupational therapists and occupational therapy assistants (AOTA, 2009b).

domain centers on helping others participate in daily life activities. The broad term that the profession uses to describe daily life activities is *occupation*. As outlined in the *Framework*, occupational therapists and occupational therapy assistants[2] work collaboratively with people, organizations, and populations (clients) to engage in everyday activities or occupations that they want and need to do in a manner that supports health and participation (see Figure 1). Using occupational engagement as both the desired outcome of intervention and the intervention itself, occupational therapy practitioners are skilled at viewing the subjective and objective aspects of performance and understanding occupation simultaneously from this dual, yet holistic, perspective. The overarching mission to support health and participation in life through engagement in occupations circumscribes the profession's domain and emphasizes the important ways in which environmental and life circumstances influence the manner in which people carry out their occupations. Key aspects of the domain of occupational therapy are defined in Figure 2.

Process

Many professions use the process of evaluating, intervening, and targeting outcomes that is outlined in the *Framework*. Occupational therapy's application of this process is made unique, however, by its focus on occupation (see Figure 3).

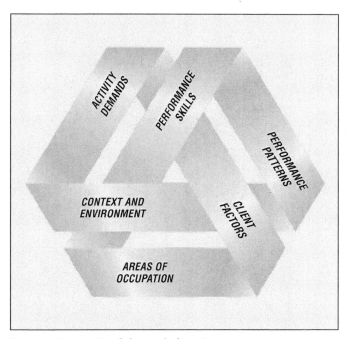

Figure 1. Occupational therapy's domain.

Reprinted from "Occupational Therapy Practice Framework: Domain and Process" (2nd ed., p. 627), by American Occupational Therapy Association, 2008, *American Journal of Occupational Theraphy, 62*, 625–683. Used with permission.

---

[2]*Occupational therapists* are responsible for all aspects of occupational therapy service delivery and are accountable for the safety and effectiveness of the occupational therapy service delivery process. *Occupational therapy assistants* deliver occupational therapy services under the supervision of and in partnership with an occupational therapist (AOTA, 2009a).

AREAS OF OCCUPATION	CLIENT FACTORS	PERFORMANCE SKILLS	PERFORMANCE PATTERNS	CONTEXT AND ENVIRONMENT	ACTIVITY DEMANDS
Activities of Daily Living (ADL)* Instrumental Activities of Daily Living (IADL) Rest and Sleep Education Work Play Leisure Social Participation *Also referred to as *basic activities of daily living (BADL)* or *personal activities of daily living (PADL).*	Values, Beliefs, and Spirituality Body Functions Body Structures	Sensory Perceptual Skills Motor and Praxis Skills Emotional Regulation Skills Cognitive Skills Communication and Social Skills	Habits Routines Roles Rituals	Cultural Personal Physical Social Temporal Virtual	Objects Used and Their Properties Space Demands Social Demands Sequencing and Timing Required Actions Required Body Functions Required Body Structures

Figure 2. Aspects of occupational therapy's domain.

Reprinted from "Occupational Therapy Practice Framework: Domain and Process" (2nd ed., p. 628), by American Occupational Therapy Association, 2008, *American Journal of Occupational Therapy, 62,* 625–683. Used with permission.

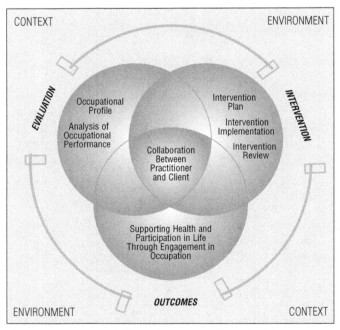

Figure 3. Occupational therapy's process of service delivery as applied within the profession's domain.

Reprinted from "Occupational Therapy Practice Framework: Domain and Process" (2nd ed., p. 627), by American Occupational Therapy Association, 2008, *American Journal of Occupational Therapy, 62,* 625–683. Used with permission.

The process of occupational therapy service delivery typically begins with the *occupational profile*—an assessment of the client's occupational needs, problems, and concerns—and the *analysis of occupational performance*, which includes the skills, patterns, contexts and environments, activity demands, and client factors that contribute to or impede the client's satisfaction with his or her ability to engage in valued daily life activities. Therapists then plan and implement intervention using a variety of approaches and methods in which occupation is both the means and ends (Trombly, 1995).

Occupational therapists continually assess the effectiveness of the intervention and the client's progress toward targeted outcomes. The intervention review informs decisions to continue or discontinue intervention and to make referrals to other agencies or professionals. Therapists select outcome measures that are valid, reliable, and appropriately sensitive to the client's occupational performance, satisfaction, adaptation, role competence, health and wellness, prevention, self-advocacy, quality of life, and *occupational justice* (i.e., access to and opportunities for participation in the full range of meaningful and enriching occupations afforded to others within the community to satisfy personal, health, and societal needs; Wilcock & Townsend, 2008).

Mental Health Promotion, Prevention, and Intervention for Children and Youth

Background

Over the years, the view of children's mental health services has changed. This change in thinking has also altered how occupational therapy services are perceived and implemented. Whereas earlier views tended to narrowly focus only on services provided to children with diagnosed mental illness provided in psychiatric settings, more recent approaches have expanded the scope of services. According to Bazyk (2011c), children's mental health also focuses on services aimed at helping children develop and maintain mental health. Using this framework, occupational therapy practitioners provide services to all children with and without identified mental health illness in school, community, and health care settings.

Explanations of the components of mental health typically include four characteristics:
1. Positive affective or emotional state (e.g., subjective sense of well-being, feeling happy)
2. Positive psychological and social function (e.g., self-acceptance, fulfilling relationships, self-control)
3. Productive activities
4. Resilience in the face of adversity and the ability to cope with life stressors (U.S. Department of Health and Human Services, 1999; WHO, 2004).

Quite simply, *positive mental health* refers to "feeling well" and "doing well" (Miles, Espiritu, Horen, Sebian, & Waetzig, 2010).

Mental ill health is an umbrella term that includes a continuum from the most severe disorders to mild symptoms of differing duration and intensity (Barry & Jenkins, 2007). The terms *mental illness* and *mental disorders* commonly are used to refer to diagnosable psychiatric conditions that significantly interfere with a person's functioning, such as bipolar disorder, schizophrenia, and dementia. *Mental health problems* often refers to more common issues, such as anxiety and depression, which may be less severe and of shorter duration but, if left unattended, may develop into more serious conditions (Barry & Jenkins, 2007).

Mental health is also perceived as a dynamic state of functioning that can vary throughout a person's life on the basis of several of biological (e.g., genetics), environmental (e.g., poverty), situational (e.g., death of a parent), or developmental factors (Barry & Jenkins, 2007). "Children's mental health, in particular, needs to be understood in a somewhat different context from adult mental health" (Miles et al., 2010, p. 21). Knowledge of development, including how it is influenced by the complex interaction among several biological, psychological, and social factors, is critical.

Developmental Factors Affecting Mental Health

Because development occurs in nested contexts of family, school, neighborhood, and the larger society, an ecological perspective of intervention is widely accepted. Understanding the pathways of development enables prevention researchers and practitioners to identify opportunities for modifying pathological developmental trajectories. Individual, family, school, and community characteristics that foster mental health development across different developmental stages are summarized in Table 1. Mental health promotion focuses on efforts to enhance the person's ability to gain such developmental competencies.

Developmental psychopathology is an integrative multidisciplinary area of study that applies a developmental approach to understanding the pathways toward or away from mental health problems and disorders in children and youth (Masten, 2006).

Table 1. Factors Associated With Positive Development and Prevention of Mental Health Problems Over Time

	Individual	Family	School & Community
Infancy and early childhood	• Secure attachment • Emotional regulation • Appropriate conduct • Making friends • Understanding self and other's emotions	• Adequate prenatal and postnatal health care • Nurturing relationship with caregiver (reliable, responsive, affectionate) • Support for the development of new skills	• Availability of high-quality child care • Support for early learning • Access to supplemental services, such as screening for vision/hearing • Low ratio of caregivers to children
Middle childhood	• Academic achievement • Appropriate behavior • Positive peer relations • Resilience (ability to adapt to life stressors) • Empathy • Satisfying friendships	• Emotionally responsive interactions with children • Consistent discipline • Language-based rather than physically based discipline • Parental resources, including positive personal efficacy and adaptive coping	• High academic standards and strong leadership • Teacher support • Effective classroom management • Positive family–school relations • School policies and practices to reduce bullying
Adolescence	• Physical health • Intellectual development • Psychological and emotional development • Social development • Connectiveness to peers, family, and community	• Physical and psychological safety • Appropriate structure (limits, rules, predictability) • Supportive relationships • Opportunities to belong • Positive social norms (expectations, values) • Opportunities for skill building • Integration of family, school, and community	• Physical and psychological safety • Appropriate structure (limits, rules, predictability) • Supportive relationships • Opportunities to belong • Positive social norms (expectations, values) • Opportunities for skill building • Integration of family, school, and community
Early adulthood	• Explore identity in love, work, and world view (e.g., values) to obtain a broad range of life experiences and move toward making commitments around which to structure adult life • Subjective sense of adult status in self-sufficiency, making independent decisions, becoming financially independent • Future orientation and achievement motivation	• Behavioral and emotional autonomy • Balance of autonomy and relatedness to family	• Opportunities for exploration in school and work • Connectiveness to adults outside of family

Source. From "Using a Developmental Framework to Guide Prevention and Promotion," in *Preventing Mental, Emotional, and Behavioral Disorders Among Young People: Progress and Possibilities* (pp. 78–80), by Mary Ellen O'Connell, Thomas Boar, and Kenneth E. Warner (Eds.), 2009, Washington, DC: National Academies Press. Copyright © 2009 by the National Academies Press. Used with permission.

Mental health development is characterized by age-related changes in several areas, including cognitive, emotional, and behavioral abilities. As children mature, successful completion of developmental tasks leads to an overall balanced view of strengths and weaknesses (Catalano, Hawkins, Berglund, Pollard, & Arthur, 2002). Competencies gained at one stage of development provide a foundation for future competencies as the young person faces new challenges and opportunities. Understanding the age-related patterns of competence and disorder is important for developing promotion and prevention interventions (National Research Council [NRC] & Institute of Medicine [IOM], 2009).

Attention to the onset of various mental health disorders is also important. For example, longitudinal studies have identified that the median age of onset for anxiety and impulse control disorders is 11 years, with substance abuse disorders occurring at age 20 and mood disorders at age 30 (Kessler et al., 2005). Research indicates that initial symptoms generally appear 2 to 4 years prior to the onset of a full-blown disorder, suggesting the importance of early screening and intervention.

The concept of *developmental cascades* refers to the interaction between problems and competencies over time (Masten et al., 2005). For example, externalizing behavioral problems (e.g., conduct disorder) leads to lower academic performance in adolescence, which leads to increased internalizing emotional problems (e.g., anxiety, depression) in young adulthood. Mental health promotion includes efforts to enhance individuals' ability to achieve developmentally appropriate tasks, whereas prevention programs aim to reduce risks at the biological, psychological, family, and community levels. Interventions might include programming to strengthen family and child protective factors or reduce risk factors (see Figure 4).

Developmental psychopathology guides prevention and intervention. "As the developmental patterning and timing of specific problems and disorders is increasingly well-known, particularly in relation to risks, protections, cascades, and progressions, it

becomes possible to intervene with increasingly strategic timing and targets" (Masten, 2006, p. 51).

Prevalence of Disorders and Impairments

The U.S. Surgeon General has estimated that between 5% and 11% of school-age children have mental health disorders that result in "extreme" or "significant" functional impairment (NRC & IOM, 2009; U.S. Department of Health and Human Services, 1999). This indicates that, of the 70 million children and adolescents in the United States, 6 million to 9 million have a serious emotional disturbance. Only 1 in 5, however, receives any professional help, indicating that a significant proportion of this population is underserved.

Risk and Protective Factors

Risk factors increase the likelihood that mental health problems will develop, and protective factors reduce the likelihood that a disorder will develop. Risk and protective factors occur at multiple levels, including the individual, family, community, and society levels. (See Table 2 for definitions of factors.) Adverse childhood experiences, which include child abuse/neglect and exposure to other traumatic stressors, commonly result in a multitude of short- and long-term emotional, physical, and social problems (Felitti et al., 1998). Because a variety of social, community, and family factors influence mental health, there have been calls for comprehensive mental health promotion and prevention programs that extend beyond an individual focus (Barry & Jenkins, 2007; WHO, 2001).

Federal Legislation and the Role of Occupational Therapy

Mental health services for children were once provided almost exclusively in hospitals and community mental health centers, but the Education

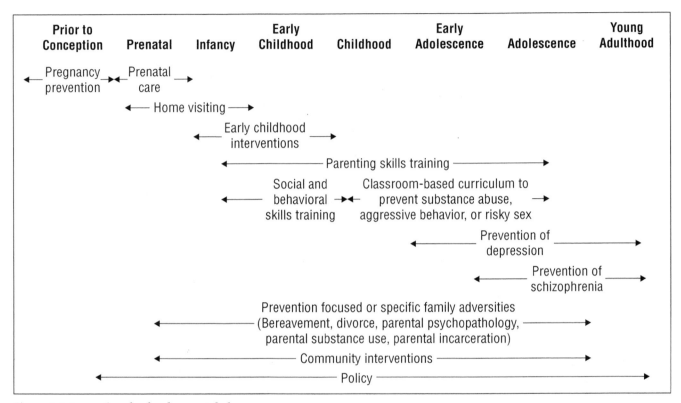

Figure 4. Interventions by developmental phase.

Source. From "Using a Developmental Framework to Guide Prevention and Promotion," in *Preventing Mental, Emotional, and Behavioral Disorders Among Young People: Progress and Possibilities* (p. 155), by Mary Ellen O'Connell, Thomas Baot, and Kenneth E. Warner (Eds.), 2009, Washington, DC: National Academies Press. Copyright © 2009 by the National Academies Press. Used with permission.

for All Handicapped Children Act of 1975 (Pub. L. 94–142)—the first federal initiative that required schools to meet the mental health needs of students with emotional disturbance—has played a key role in blurring the lines of responsibility for where such services should be provided (Bazyk, 2007; Kutash, Duchnowski, & Lynn, 2006). However, because the Individuals with Disabilities Education Act of 1997 (IDEA 1997; Pub. L. 105–117) focuses solely on students with identifiable disabilities that interfere with academic achievement, only a small percentage of children needing mental health services are guaranteed such care in school under IDEA. Nonetheless, now most children receiving mental health services obtain this care in schools, making schools the "de facto mental health system for children in this country" (Kutash et al., 2006, p. 62).

IDEA 1997 placed greater emphasis on the inclusion of students with disabilities in general education by embedding special education and related services in the classroom and extracurricular activities when possible. General and special education practices have further aligned as a result of the Individuals with Disabilities Education Improvement Act of 2004 (IDEA 2004; Pub. L. 108–446) and the No Child Left Behind Act of 2001 (Pub. L. 107–110), providing school personnel, including occupational therapists, with increasing opportunities to expand their role in schools, in particular in the area of prevention (Cahill, 2007).

Mental Health Promotion, Prevention, and Intervention for Children and Youth

Table 2. Risk and Protective Factors Associated With Positive Mental Health

	Protective Factors	Risk Factors
Individual	• Positive sense of self • Good physical health • Effective social skills • Close relationship to family • Good coping skills	• Low self-esteem • Chronic illness or physical disability • Poor social skills • Insecure attachment to family • Poor coping skills
Social	• Caring and supportive parents • Positive early attachment • Sense of social belonging • Supportive relationships • Participation in the community	• Social isolation • Abuse, neglect, and/or violence • Peer rejection • Separation and loss
Systems	• Safe living environment • Economic security • Positive educational experience • Access to health and other supports	• Neighborhood violence and crime • Poverty • Unemployment • Homelessness • School failure • Lack of health and other support services

Source. From *Implementing Mental Health Promotion* (p. 6), by Margaret M. Barry & Rachel Jenkins, 2007, Edinburgh, Scotland: Churchill Livingston/Elsevier. Copyright © 2007 by Elsevier. Adapted with permission.

Another shift is likely to take place for children who are newly insured under provisions of the Patient Protection and Affordable Care Act of 2010 (Pub. L. 111–148), because most of the newly insured population will be enrolled in plans that are required to cover mental and behavioral health intervention as "essential health benefits."

A national movement to develop and expand school mental health services has grown during the past two decades as a result of the high prevalence of mental health needs among youth and the awareness that more youth can be reached in schools (Masia-Warner, Nangle, & Hansen, 2006; Weist & Paternite, 2006). Prominent federal initiatives (President's New Freedom Commission on Mental Health, 2003; U. S. Department of Health and Human Services, 1999) have identified gaps in services, forcing federal, state, and local child-serving agencies to address the mental health needs of children attending school (Weist & Paternite, 2006).

Schools must be active partners in the mental health of children because it is currently accepted that a major barrier to learning is immature or limited social–emotional skills and not necessarily cognitive impairment (Koller & Bertel, 2006). School mental health can be thought of as a framework of approaches expanding on traditional methods to promote children's mental health by emphasizing prevention, positive youth development, and schoolwide approaches (see http://www.schoolmentalhealth.org/resources/esmh/defesmh.html). This school mental health framework promotes interdisciplinary collaboration among mental health providers, related service providers, teachers, and school administrators to meet the mental health needs of all students.

Legislative changes also have prompted schools to shift to a multitiered model of services committing to the success of all students by providing early identification and early intervening services. The reauthorization of IDEA in 1997 began to erode the traditional thinking that special education and general education are separate programs serving separate populations (Spencer, Turkett, Vaughan, & Koenig, 2006). IDEA 1997 placed greater emphasis on the inclusion of students with disabilities in general education by embedding special education and related services in the classroom and extracurricular activities when possible. In addition to school legislation, occupational therapy for children is also mandated under Medicaid—Early Periodic Screening, Diagnosis and Treatment.

The field of occupational therapy is well positioned to provide services to children and youth with behavioral and psychosocial needs and their families, in particular in educational settings. The psychosocial dimension of human performance is fundamental to all aspects of occupational therapy with every client population and in all practice settings. Occupational therapy values the dynamic and interactive relationship between the client and his or her performance skills, the demands of the activity, and the physical and social contexts within which the activity is performed.

Interruption in a person's ability to engage in and succeed at necessary and valued occupations elicits emotional and psychological responses that are central to how the person responds and eventually adapts. Occupational therapists understand both the observable and unobservable aspects of an individual's performance and take them into account when performing the occupation-based evaluation and identifying relevant outcomes and effective interventions (Kannenberg & Greene, 2003). Occupational therapy practitioners are prepared to intervene on multiple levels: with individual children and their families, on their behalf at the institution and community levels, and in the realm of policy formation.

A Public Health Approach to Children's Mental Health

The mission of public health is to fulfill society's interest in making sure that conditions exist in which people can be healthy (IOM, Committee for the Study of the Future of Public Health, Division of Health Care Services, 1988). This is accomplished by "collaborating to create the expertise, information and tools that people and communities need to protect their health— through health promotion, prevention of disease, injury and disability, and preparedness for new health threats" (see http://www.cdc.gov/about /organization/mission.htm). Given the previously described perspective of mental health, WHO (2001) has advocated a public health approach to mental health that emphasizes the promotion of mental health as well as the prevention of and intervention for mental illness. National leaders in the field of children's mental health also have promoted the adoption of a public health approach to children's mental health in recent high-profile publications and other resources (Atkins, Hoagwood, Kutash, & Seidman, 2010; Barry & Jenkins, 2007; Bershad & Blaber, 2011; Miles et al., 2010; Stiffman et al., 2010; Substance Abuse and Mental Health Services Administration, 2012).

Although occupational therapy has a rich history of promoting mental health in all areas of practice, reference to *children's mental health* has traditionally been interpreted to mean intervention to prevent and/or treat mental health problems (Davidson, 2005; Lougher, 2001). The more recent interpretation of children's mental health has broadened to address the needs of all children through promotion and prevention of, in addition to intervention in, mental illness (AOTA, 2010a, 2010b; Bazyk, 2011c).

Positive mental health is considered fundamental to overall health and quality of life and contributes to the functioning of individuals, families, communities, and societies (Barry & Jenkins, 2007). As such, mental health can be located within a health promotion framework, which is based on an empowering, participative, and collaborative process to help people take control of and improve their health (WHO, 1986). Barry and Jenkins (2007) applied this framework to the promotion of mental health in the following five areas: (a) building healthy public policy, (b) creating supportive environments, (c) strengthening community action, (d) developing personal skills, and (e) reorienting health services (see Box 1).

Box 1. Socioecological Framework for Mental Health Promotion

The Ottawa Charter for Health Promotion (World Health Organization, 1986) outlines the following five areas as important for mental health promotion:

1. *Building healthy public policy:* Calls all policymakers to put mental health promotion on the agenda to foster coordinated action across health, economic, and social policies to improve mental health. Policies related to employment, housing, education, and child care, for example, are viewed as affecting the mental health of the whole population.

2. *Creating supportive environments:* Focuses on the interaction between people and their environments, including the social, physical, cultural, and economic aspects of the environment. Key contexts for creating and promoting positive mental health include homes, schools, workplaces, and community settings. *Examples:* Promote mental health in schools; reduce disadvantage and prevent stigma.

3. *Strengthening community action:* Emphasizes the empowerment of communities through active efforts to identify their own needs, set priorities, and plan and implement action to promote optimal health. Community development approaches promote public participation and increased capacity to improve mental health at the community level.

4. *Developing personal skills:* Involves promoting personal and social development by providing information, education, and skill training. Information and education to foster mental health literacy can target schools and families so that children and youth understand positive mental health as an integral part of overall health. *Examples:* Teach children about positive mental health in schools; educate parents on how to foster mental health in their children.

5. *Reorienting health services:* Calls for mental health services that emphasize promotion and prevention activities and the treatment of mental illness across a variety of groups, for example, children, young mothers, and people with chronic health problems, disabilities, or both. Reorienting health services to promote mental health requires greater attention to education of health care providers and reorganization of health services.

Source. From *Implementing Mental Health Promotion* (p. 16), by Margaret M. Barry and Rachel Jenkins, 2007, Edinburgh, Scotland: Churchill Livingstone/Elsevier. Copyright © 2007 by Elsevier. Adapted with permission.

The Occupational Therapy Process: Applying a Public Health Approach to Mental Health in Children and Youth

A public health model is presented in this Practice Guideline to envision and guide occupational therapy services in the promotion of mental health and prevention and intervention of mental ill health for school, community, and health care settings. This framework supports a change in thinking from the traditional individually focused, deficit-driven model of mental health intervention to a whole-population, strengths-based approach.

Populations and Settings

Such a shift in thinking requires careful reflection on several questions related to *whom* occupational therapy should serve, and *where*, followed by a strategic conceptualization of *what* occupational therapy services might entail. In terms of *whom*, when adopting a public health approach to mental health, occupational therapy practitioners can serve *all* children—both those with and without disabilities and mental health disorders.

Although services can be offered in a variety of settings—school, health care, and community settings are prominent contexts for the provision of occupational therapy services for children and youth and are emphasized in this Practice Guideline. Although the domain and process of our services will be similar in each setting, the focus will differ. For example, in schools, the role of occupational therapy is to help children benefit from their education and function successfully in the school environment. In contrast, services provided in the community likely will occur during out-of-school time, warranting attention to the development of meaningful, structured leisure interests, friendships, independent living skills, and beginning work skills.

Occupation-Based Practice

In terms of *what* our services entail, although the emphasis of occupational therapy will vary depending on context, all efforts share a common belief in the positive relationship between participation in a balance of meaningful occupations and health. Although the second edition of the *Framework* is not considered a theory or model, it provides a useful tool for framing occupational therapy practice and is applied throughout this Practice Guideline to describe occupational therapy services. In combination, the domain and process of occupational therapy guide practitioners in promoting *occupational performance*—which results from the dynamic intersection of the client, context, and occupation (AOTA, 2008). This ecological model, which reflects a longstanding and prominent understanding of the relationship among person, occupation, and environment, has been described from numerous perspectives both within and outside of occupational therapy (Dunn, Brown, & Youngstrom, 2003; Law et al., 1996; Rogers & Holm, 2009).

Just as factors within the person may support or impede occupational performance, so too can the environment have a positive or negative influence. A core skill for all occupational therapy practitioners is *activity analysis:* the ability to analyze the relationship among the person, environment, and activity and determine factors needed for successful participation. When the task environment demands are greater than the person's abilities, the intervention may involve increasing/developing the skill and/or adaptating the environment or the task to foster successful participation (Rogers & Holm, 2009). The therapeutic use of occupation is used as a means to bring about occupational performance.

Although several approaches specific to mental health promotion are important to know about and apply, all occupational therapy services share a common emphasis on the use of meaningful occupation to promote occupational performance (education, play, leisure, work, social participation, activities of daily living [ADLs], instrumental activities of daily living, sleep/rest within a variety of contexts; AOTA, 2008). There are seemingly endless opportunities for using occupation-based strategies in school, home, and community settings to promote mental health, because all occupational therapy services emphasize competency enhancement. In schools, occupation-based services can be embedded in several natural contexts, including academic classrooms, the cafeteria (lunch groups), recess (game clubs), art, and physical education. Increased emphasis is being placed on participation in extracurricular activities, opening doors for occupational therapy practitioners to help children and youth develop and participate in structured leisure interests during after-school hours. Participation in a variety of community-based activities, including the arts, recreation, music, sports, or club activities, can be promoted using coaching strategies.

Interventions

Within a public health model of mental health, the three major levels of service include

1. The *universal* or whole population,
2. *Targeted* or selective services, and
3. *Intensive* services (see Figure 5).

Although interventions are provided at each level, the focus will vary. According to the *Framework*, the intervention process consists of skilled action taken by occupational therapy practitioners in collaboration with the client (person, population, community) to foster engagement in occupation related to health and participation (AOTA, 2008).

Leaders in the field of mental health promotion and prevention also use the term *intervention* to describe their efforts (Miles et al., 2010; NRC & IOM, 2009). In this Practice Guideline, *intervention* is defined broadly to refer to a variety of services (promotion, prevention, intensive) that are provided within the tiers that create positive changes in the mental health of children and youth at the individual, group, subpopulation, or population level (AOTA, 2008; Miles et al., 2010).

A variety of intervention approaches are available from within and outside of the field of occupational therapy that can be used to address performance skills by reducing symptoms, minimizing risks, and building competencies specific to children's mental health. This Practice Guideline presents several approaches that are useful in minimizing mental health problems and building competencies within the domain of occupational

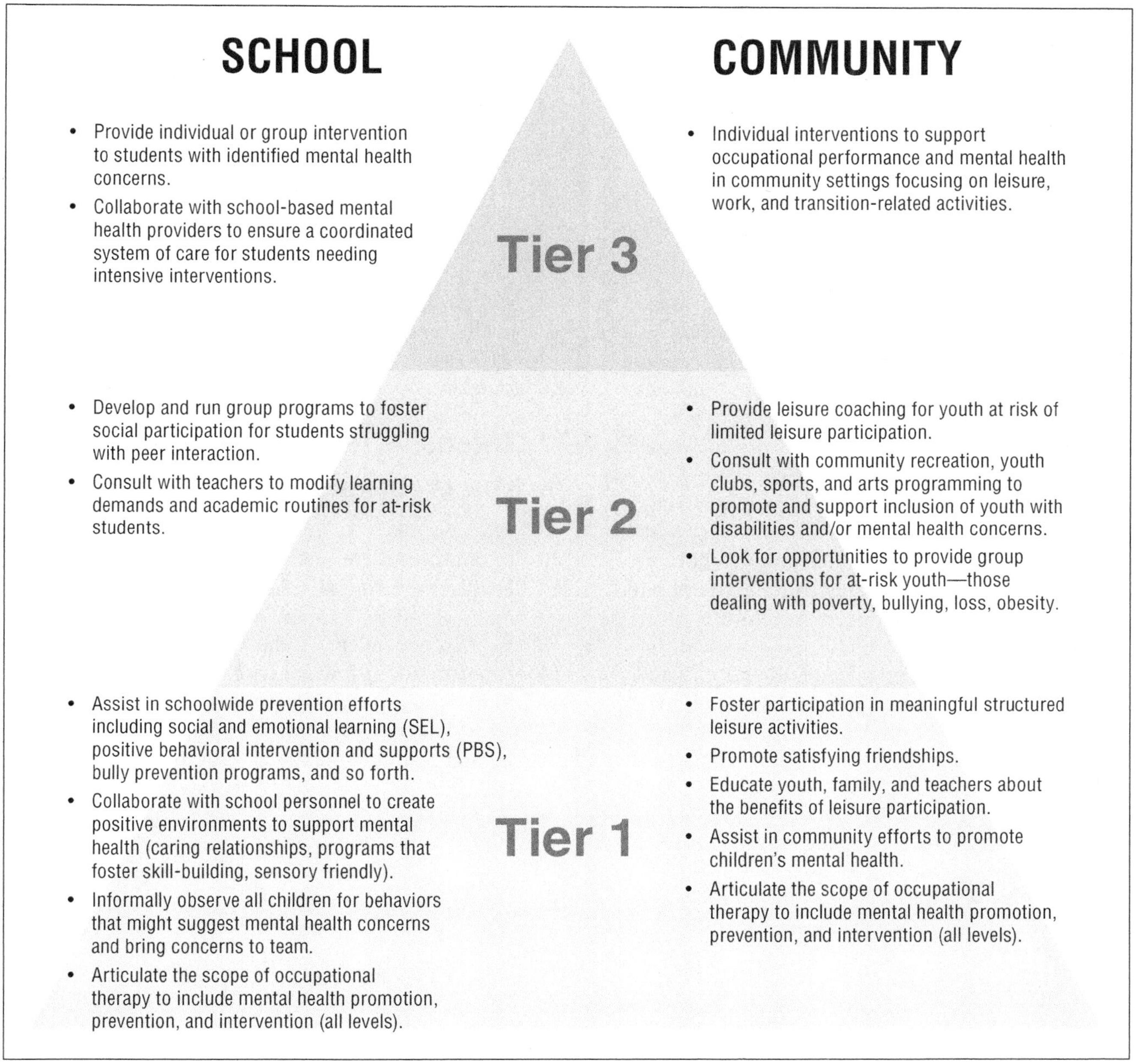

SCHOOL

Tier 3

- Provide individual or group intervention to students with identified mental health concerns.
- Collaborate with school-based mental health providers to ensure a coordinated system of care for students needing intensive interventions.

Tier 2

- Develop and run group programs to foster social participation for students struggling with peer interaction.
- Consult with teachers to modify learning demands and academic routines for at-risk students.

Tier 1

- Assist in schoolwide prevention efforts including social and emotional learning (SEL), positive behavioral intervention and supports (PBS), bully prevention programs, and so forth.
- Collaborate with school personnel to create positive environments to support mental health (caring relationships, programs that foster skill-building, sensory friendly).
- Informally observe all children for behaviors that might suggest mental health concerns and bring concerns to team.
- Articulate the scope of occupational therapy to include mental health promotion, prevention, and intervention (all levels).

COMMUNITY

Tier 3

- Individual interventions to support occupational performance and mental health in community settings focusing on leisure, work, and transition-related activities.

Tier 2

- Provide leisure coaching for youth at risk of limited leisure participation.
- Consult with community recreation, youth clubs, sports, and arts programming to promote and support inclusion of youth with disabilities and/or mental health concerns.
- Look for opportunities to provide group interventions for at-risk youth—those dealing with poverty, bullying, loss, obesity.

Tier 1

- Foster participation in meaningful structured leisure activities.
- Promote satisfying friendships.
- Educate youth, family, and teachers about the benefits of leisure participation.
- Assist in community efforts to promote children's mental health.
- Articulate the scope of occupational therapy to include mental health promotion, prevention, and intervention (all levels).

Figure 5. School and community tiers.

therapy practice. The intent is not to provide fully comprehensive and complete information on all possible approaches but to provide foundation information, strategies for implementation, and useful resources for further learning.

Promotion Interventions

Because a public health approach to mental health involves promotion, prevention, and intensive interventions, it is important to make distinctions among these practices. *Mental health promotion interventions focus on competence enhancement* — on building strengths and resources in the whole population (Barry & Jenkins, 2007). As such, this framework emphasizes optimizing health by improving the social, physical, and economic environments that determine the mental health of individuals and populations (Miles et al., 2010). Mental health promotion, while addressing the needs of the whole population, also addresses the needs of those experiencing mental ill health, which includes creating supportive environments, reducing stigma and discrimination, and supporting the social and emotional health of clients and their families (Barry & Jenkins, 2007).

Prevention Interventions

Prevention interventions were developed over the past two decades and have traditionally focused on reducing the incidence and seriousness of problem behaviors and mental health disorders (Barry & Jenkins, 2007; Catalano et al., 2002). Early prevention programs tended to focus primarily on *reducing risk factors* (e.g., family history of substance abuse, poverty); however, current approaches recognize the importance of minimizing mental health problems by enhancing protective factors as well (e.g., social and emotional competencies, clear standards for behavior; Miles et al., 2010).

Intensive Individualized Interventions

Intensive individualized interventions are provided to diminish the effects of an identified mental health problem and restore the child to an optimal state of functioning. Intervention at this level is often dependent on the specific mental health problem and/or formal diagnosis. In addition to diminishing problems at this level, it is critical to also focus on promoting or optimizing positive mental health (Miles et al., 2010).

Three Major Tiers of Service

The occupational therapy process described in the following sections clearly differentiates service provision for each tier specific to evaluation and intervention.

Tier 1: Universal Mental Health Promotion and Prevention Services

Services at this level are geared toward the entire population, including children and youth with or without mental health or behavioral problems, as well as with other disabilities and illnesses. At the universal level, the occupational therapy process focuses less on direct, individualized care and more on indirect services geared toward groups of children and youth.

Evaluation

Evaluation occurs at a broad institutional or community level. On the basis of a sound awareness of best practice related to mental health promotion and prevention, occupational therapy practitioners should evaluate school and community settings for the presence and quality of such efforts. As mentioned earlier, the occupational profile consists of obtaining information about schoolwide and community-based promotion and prevention initiatives such as social and emotional learning (SEL) and positive behavioral intervention and supports (PBS; discussed below).

It is important that occupational therapy practitioners assist school teams in implementing

such whole-school approaches. Evaluation also should include attention to children and youths' emotions as they participate in occupations that they need or want to do. Does the physical and social environment support successful participation and enjoyment? If not, what accommodations and or adaptations, based on an analysis of person–occupation–environment, might the occupational therapy practitioner offer? For example, how does the school cafeteria support positive social interaction and successful participation in the mealtime occupation? Is recess organized in a way to promote age-appropriate play and social participation? How is positive behavior fostered in school hallways, classrooms, restrooms, and on the bus? What settings in the community offer inclusive opportunities for participation in sports, dance, music, or creative arts programming?

In addition, it is important to become knowledgeable about key legislation and policies that influence mental health promotion and prevention efforts. For example, the President's New Freedom Commission on Mental Health (2003) identified fragmentation and gaps in care and specifically recommended that all federal, state, and local child-serving agencies address the mental health needs of youth in the educational system (see also Weist & Paternite, 2006). The commission "emphasized building a mental health system that is evidence-based, recovery-focused and consumer- and family-driven" (Moherek Sopko, 2006, p. 1). Last, it is critical to become familiar with reputable technical assistance centers in order to develop and maintain information related to mental health promotion (see Box 2).

Box 2. Internet Resources on Mental Health

Federal Government
- *Substance Abuse and Mental Health Services Administration (SAMHSA):* "Caring for Every Child's Mental Health" is a public awareness initiative that host an annual National Children's Mental Health Awareness Day event each May to raise awareness about the importance of positive mental health as an essential aspect of healthy development.
  www.samhsa.gov/children
- *National Institute of Mental Health (NIMH):* NIMH's mission is to diminish the burden of mental illness through research.
  www.nimh.nih.gov
- *Office of the U.S. Surgeon General:* In 1999, Surgeon General David Satcher issued a comprehensive report on mental health; Chapter 3 covers children and adolescents.
  http://profiles.nlm.nih.gov/ps/retrieve/Resource/Metadata/NNBBHS

Advocacy Organizations and Technical Assistance Centers
- *Bazelon Center for Mental Health Law:* The Bazelon Center works on a broad array of children's mental health issues.
  www.bazelon.org
- *National Alliance on Mental Illness (NAMI):* NAMI is the nation's largest grassroots mental health organization dedicated to improving the lives of children and adults living with mental illness and their families. Founded in 1979, NAMI has become the nation's voice on mental illness—a national organization that includes NAMI organizations in every state and in more than 1,100 local communities across the country who join together to meet the NAMI mission through advocacy, research, support, and education.
  www.nami.org
- *Centers for School Mental Health—Technical Assistance Centers:* In 1995, two national training and technical assistance centers focused on mental health in schools were established with partial support from the U.S. Department of Health and Human Services and the Center for Mental Health Services. One center is at the University of California, Los Angeles, and the other is at the University of Maryland at Baltimore. Their Web sites include information and resources on school-based mental health programs.
  www.smhp.psych.ucla.edu
  Center for School Mental Health
  www.csmh.umaryland.edu
  Center for Mental Health in Schools
- *Minnesota Association for Children's Mental Health:* The association offers practical school mental health resources based on current research and effective programming.
  - Early Childhood Fact Sheets cover a range of conditions (depression, sensory processing disorders) and offer information for parents on such topics as tantrums and toileting.
  - Mental Health Fact Sheets provide information about a variety of conditions (e.g., anxiety disorders, schizophrenia), symptoms, educational implications, instructional strategies, and classroom accommodations.
  www.macmh.org

(Continued)

Intervention

Intervention emphasizes supporting whole-school or community-based approaches that foster positive mental health and well-being in all children. At this level, it is critical for occupational therapy practitioners to work collaboratively with a wide variety of individuals, including administrators, teachers, health educators, school nurses, social workers, and families. It is important first to identify what educational policies and established programs exist so that systematic efforts can be made to ensure that an occupational therapist becomes an active and recognized team member within these systems of care. Because at least 80% of the team needs to buy into new approaches to ensure successful implementation, it is critical that all members of the school team (including occupational therapists) be involved in schoolwide training efforts and actively assist in program implementation (Kutash et al., 2006).

Universal services reflect a dual commitment to promotion (development of competencies and positive mental health) and prevention (reduction of risks) in the whole population, including the majority of children who do not demonstrate academic or emotional problems. Research suggests that focusing on both risk reduction and protective factor enhancement is most effective in promoting positive youth development (Catalano et al., 2002; Mrazek & Haggerty, 1994). Within multiple settings, occupational therapy practitioners have numerous opportunities to build competencies and reduce risks in children and youth. A key to moving in this direction is being committed to such efforts and actively seeking opportunities to practice in such a manner.

Approaches Emphasizing Mental Health Promotion

Promotion efforts focus on competence enhancement and positive mental health in the whole population within the context of their everyday lives. Such an enhancement model assumes that, as children become more competent, their psychological well-being improves (Barry & Jenkins, 2007). All children can benefit from home, school, and community resources that help in the development of personal and social skills (e.g., coping, self-awareness, emotion regulation).

Promotion efforts need to involve a comprehensive life span approach that takes into consideration the age-, situation-, group-, and society-related determinants of and impediments to mental health and wellness. According to Cowen (1991), comprehensive promotion efforts should focus on four areas: (1) competence (social–emotional, leisure, and work skills), (2) resilience (ability to cope with life stressors), (3) social system modification (changing social environments to promote mental health), and (4) empowerment (enhancing children's control over their mental health). Occupational therapists have ample opportunities to promote positive mental health given that their services, through the use of meaningful occupations, foster the development of needed and desired occupations.

However, in schools, promotion efforts are traditionally restricted to a few children: those with identified disabilities, not the whole population. This, in part, is influenced by restrictions within the setting (e.g., in most schools, children must be "eligible" for special education and related services) and those imparted by insurance companies. So, although occupational therapy practitioners are well equipped to provide services to promote mental health and well-being in the whole population, social system modifications are needed to support this shift in service provision.

It is essential that occupational therapists look for opportunities to expand services to include mental health promotion and advocate for such shifts in service delivery. Occupational therapy practitioners' job expectations within school settings have traditionally been based on a *caseload* model of counting the number of children receiving direct intervention as a part of their individualized education program (IEP; AOTA, 2006). This model often neglects to account for essential indirect services, including collaborative consultation, team meetings, and in-service trainings. In contrast, the concept of *workload* encompasses all of the direct and indirect services performed to benefit students, making a workload approach helpful for conceptualizing work patterns that optimize effectiveness and impact (AOTA, 2006).

Recent efforts to prevent school failure in IDEA 2004 included response to intervention (RtI) as a framework for early identification and intervention for academic and behavior problems (AOTA, 2006). Similarly, schoolwide PBS supports all students along a continuum of need based on the three-tiered prevention model. These approaches provide a mechanism to address behavioral and/or academic challenges without the requirement of an IEP. Finally, "an important component of integrating mental health efforts into the ongoing routines of schools is the identification and support of indigenous persons and resources within schools as agents of change" (Atkins et al., 2010, p. 42). Occupational therapy practitioners, with their professional background in mental health, should function as such indigenous resources for integrating mental health efforts in schools.

As a schoolwide universal service, occupational therapy practitioners might collaborate with health educators or school nurses in co-teaching a unit on the mental health continuum, including mental illness, moderate mental health, and flourishing (Keyes, 2007). Programs that help children learn and talk about mental health, mental illness, and interventions may help reduce the negative stigma associated with mental illness by helping bring the topic into everyday conversations and framing mental health as a positive state of functioning (Jorm, 2012). Becoming aware of and encouraging use of reliable Internet resources is another strategy for promoting mental health literacy. Santor and colleagues (Santor, Poulin, Leblanc, & Kususmakar, 2007) has developed and explored the use and impact of a school-based health information Web site for adolescents. Their findings indicated that the use of such a Web site holds promise for health promotion and early self-identification for emotional problems.

There are multiple programs and approaches applied in schools and the community that focus on the promotion of mental health; SEL, PBS, and participation in structured leisure activities are described in the following sections. Other options, such as mental health literacy and sensory processing, are discussed in Appendix D.

Social and emotional learning. Developed as a conceptual framework in 1994 to focus on the emotional needs of children and address the fragmented programs meant to address those needs (Greenberg et al., 2003), *SEL* is defined as a process for helping children develop critical skills for life effectiveness, including developing positive relationships, behaving ethically, and handling challenging situations effectively (Collaborative for Academic, Social, and Emotional Learning [CASEL], 2009). Specifically, programs that foster SEL help children recognize and manage emotions, think about their feelings and how one should act, regulate behavior based on thoughtful decision making, and acquire important social skills for developing healthy relationships in life (Elias et al., 1997; Goleman, 1995). In other words, emotional and social skills must be developed to prevent feelings from "hijacking" thoughts and actions (Goleman, 1995).

The five major skill areas viewed as essential are (1) self-awareness, (2) self-management, (3) social awareness, (4) relationship skills, and (5) responsible decision making (CASEL, 2009). Emotional learning "lessons" should be given in small doses and delivered regularly over a sustained period of time. Experiences that are repeated allow the new skills to become neural habits that can be applied during periods of stress (Goleman, 1995). Elias and colleagues (1997) suggested that children need to develop skills in emotion, thinking, and behavior in the following four domains: (1) life skills and social competencies; (2) health promotion and problem-prevention skills; (3) coping skills and social support for transitions and crises; and (4) positive, contributory service.

SEL has grown significantly in its application throughout the United States in both school and after-school settings. As such, it is important for occupational therapy practitioners to

- Become knowledgeable about SEL and its implementation (e.g., read CASEL training materials);
- Determine whether the local school district or state has adopted SEL standards or a SEL curriculum, obtain information about such initiatives, and assist in implementation;
- Identify school committees that may address SEL programming and volunteer to become a member; and

- Embed SEL strategies into occupational therapy services (group, individual and consultative).

Although there are multiple ways to promote SEL and embed strategies within occupational therapy, being vigilant to opportunities to become a part of SEL initiatives in school or community settings is essential. Box 3 provides a vignette that demonstrates how one occupational therapist became involved in a school district's SEL initiative.

Positive behavioral interventions and supports. Behavior management has traditionally focused on changing the behaviors of children demonstrating problems (Mu & Gabriel, 2001). Recent approaches, however, focus more broadly on promoting positive behavior by considering the combined influence of multiple systems (person, classroom, school, family, and community; Sugai et al., 2000). PBS recognizes that several relevant factors can influence behavior, including those existing within the person as well as those reflected in the interaction between the child and the environment: "PBS interventions are designed to be proactive, to prevent problem behavior by altering a situation before problems escalate, and to concurrently teach appropriate alternatives" (Carr et al., 2002, as cited in Safran & Oswald, 2003, p. 361).

Recently, PBS has been applied broadly as a behaviorally based systems approach to enhance the capacity of schools, families, and communities to design effective school environments based on research-validated practices (OSEP Technical Assistance Center on Positive Behavioral Interventions and Supports, 2010). Schoolwide positive behavior support (SWPBS) systems support all students along a continuum of need based on the three-tiered PBS prevention model of (1) *universal* (all students, ~80%), (2) *selective* (students at risk for behavior problems, ~15%), and (3) *intensive* (students with chronic/intense problem behavior, ~5%; Kutash et al., 2006). It is important for occupational therapy practitioners to consider how to embed their services within each level of intervention. The Technical Assistance

Box 3. Tier 1 Universal Services: An Occupational Therapist's Contribution to Schoolwide SEL Programming

The large urban school district in which I am employed and the community it serves responded to a tragic act of violence in one of its premier high schools by conducting a full, districtwide appraisal of conditions for learning and programming that addresses safety and mental health services in the school setting.

I became aware of the resulting recommendations and preliminary implementation plan through an e-mail sent to update faculty and staff. I requested more information from the Chief Academic Officer in my district, indicating that I was in the process of completing my doctoral project, which focused on SEL and its impact on social acceptance and participation of students with autism in general education settings. I was quickly invited to become a member of the District Action Committee, which comprised primarily administrators and leaders of the teachers' and staff unions. This collaborative group's charge was to identify barriers to implementation and problem-solve "doable" solutions. I also volunteered to participate on the Evidence-Based Practice/Programs Task Force to address SEL with school district staff as well as community mental health agencies. Its charge was to review SEL curricula and recommend those that would best meet the diverse needs of our large urban school district and the unique challenges our students and families face.

As a staff occupational therapist, I have recognized over the past 21 years that students with special needs respond best to inclusion settings in which the teacher and classroom personnel consistently provide instruction in and reinforcement of social–emotional competencies. My scholarly research and experience as a school-based therapist provided a unique perspective from which to appraise curricula and learning materials to identify curricula that would be readily accessible to both general and special education students. My training and background provided a good foundation to identify key elements needed to support buy-in and sustainability of the Tier 1 SEL interventions across the district.

Based on a recent Level I meta-analysis (Durlak, Weissberg, Dymnicki, Taylor, & Schellinger, 2011), when comparing universal whole-school SEL programs with controls, students in the intervention group demonstrated significantly improved social and emotional skills along with improved behavior, academic performance, and attitudes. The District Action Committee and Evidence-Based Practice/Programs Task Force decided to implement the PATHS (Promoting Alternative Thinking Strategies) SEL curriculum in all elementary schools for grades K–5. During the spring and summer of 2011, the Collaborative for Academic Social, and Emotional Learning's (CASEL's) district consultants provided training to more than 300 building administrators, student support staff, and district leadership team members to develop district-wide understanding of social and emotional learning. The staff, in collaboration with CASEL district consultants, have developed a draft scope and sequence that incorporates SEL into the core academic disciplines.

This collaborative work of community and school leaders in my school setting has resulted in a model for improving academic achievement that recognizes that Tier 1 and Tier 2 interventions must include both academic and social–emotional conditions for learning. As occupational therapists, I believe we bring a special understanding and perspective to how the social–emotional environment impacts positive participation and performance in the school setting.

Note. From "Major Approaches Useful in Addressing the Mental Health Needs of Children and Youth: Minimizing Risks, Reducing Symptoms, and Buildng Competencies" by S. Bazyk and S. Brandenburger Shasby, in *Mental Health Promotion, Prevention, and Intervention With Children and Youth: A Guiding Framework for Occupational Therapy* (pp. 45–70), by S. Bazyk (Ed.), 2011, Bethesda, MD: AOTA Press. Copyright © 2011 by the American Occupational Therapy Association. Adapted with permission.

For further information, see http://casel.org/collaborating-districts-initiative/cleveland-ohio/ as well as the following sources: DeMar (1997), Durlak et al. (2010), Kraag et al. (2006), Lefebvre-Pinard & Reid (1980), McMahon et al. (2000), Mulcahy & Schachter (1982), Serna et al. (2000), Stevahn et al. (2000), Tankersley et al. (1996), Ttofi & Farrington (2009), Tuttle et al. (2006), Vaughan & Ridley (1983), Vreeman & Carroll (2007), and Walker et al. (1998).

Center on Positive Behavioral Interventions and Supports, established by the Office of Special Education Programs, U.S. Department of Education, provides capacity-building information and technical assistance for identifying, adapting, and sustaining effective schoolwide disciplinary practices.

SWPBS, or universal interventions, are proactively designed to create positive school environments for all students, including the majority who do not frequently present behavior problems but would benefit from incentives that motivate them to follow the school rules. Both the prevention of behavior problems and teaching positive social behaviors are emphasized for the entire school (Freeman et al., 2006).

Because implementation requires several changes at a systems level, administrative involvement and ongoing support are essential to ensure success. Other key features of SWPBS include clearly defined and communicated behavioral expectations written in positive terms (e.g., be respectful of yourself and others); specific strategies for teaching appropriate behaviors; consistent application of procedures for correcting misbehavior, including consequences; acknowledgment of appropriate behaviors; and a support plan to meet the needs of students with chronic, challenging behaviors. A majority of school staff, typically about 80%, must agree to implement the intervention, and training and support must be provided on an ongoing basis (Kutash et al., 2006).

Schools that have reported success in implementing SWPBS have identified the following benefits: increased student attendance, student and teacher self-reports of a more positive and calm environment, and reduction in the numbers of behavioral disruptions (OSEP Technical Assistance Center on Positive Behavioral Interventions and Supports, 2010).

Like schoolwide management, effective classroom management must be based on clearly stated behavioral expectations and positive learning environments (Cartledge, 2003). *Classroom management* can be defined as "actions taken by the teacher to establish order, engage students, or elicit their cooperation" (Emmer & Stough, 2001, p. 103). Occupational therapists can work collaboratively with teachers to implement PBS strategies in order to help promote positive behaviors in the classroom.

It is also important to apply PBS in nonclassroom school settings. Hallways, cafeterias, and playgrounds account for approximately 50% of all problem behaviors (Safran & Oswald, 2003). These areas typically lack routines and clear behavioral expectation.

Precorrection, active supervision, and group contingencies all have been found to be beneficial, especially when applied in combination. *Precorrection* involves adult prompts reminding students about appropriate behavior prior to a particular transition (e.g., change of classes) or activity (e.g., recess, field trip). For example, a teacher might review school rules and appropriate social behaviors for the playground. *Active supervision* involves the dynamic presence of school personnel during nonclassroom activities and is associated with fewer problem behaviors. *Group contingencies* involve rewarding the whole group of students with special snacks or activities following positive behavior (Safran & Oswald, 2003).

Participation in structured leisure activities.
An important aspect of occupation-based practice when working with children and youth is attention to the development of structured leisure participation during out-of-school time. Youth participation in structured leisure such as sports teams, clubs, and lessons is relatively common, with approximately 6 in 10 youth participating in organized out-of-school activities at any given time (Mahoney, Harris, & Eccles, 2008; Mahoney, Larson, Eccles, & Lord, 2005).

Highly structured leisure activities are associated with regular participation schedules, rule-guided interaction, direction by one or more adult leaders, an emphasis on skill development that increases in complexity and challenge, and performance that requires sustained active attention and the provision of feedback (Mahoney et al., 2005). A committee of scholars appointed by the NRC and IOM identified eight key features of contexts as promoting positive youth development: (1) physical and psychological safety; (2) appropriate structure; (3) supportive relationships; (4) opportunities for belonging; (5) positive social norms; (6) support for efficacy and mattering; (7) opportunities for skill building; and (8) integration of family, school, and community efforts (Eccles & Gootman, 2002). Although many organized leisure activities incorporate several, if not all, of these features, occupational therapy practitioners can screen and advocate for such features in youth programming.

Correlational research has demonstrated a positive relationship between participation in structured leisure and positive outcomes such as diminished delinquency, greater achievement, and increased self-efficacy and self-control (Larson, 2000). Research that used youth inventories of participation and a qualitative study that used focus groups yielded similar findings—that participation in structured leisure is associated with both personal and interpersonal development (Dworkin, Larson, & Hansen, 2003; Hansen, Larson, & Dworkin, 2003). Additional information regarding the benefits of participation in structured leisure activities can be found in Appendix D.

Approaches Emphasizing the Prevention of Mental Health Problems

Prevention efforts generally focus on risk reduction: interrupting the processes that lead to a single problem behavior (e.g., drug use, bullying, teenage pregnancy, delinquent behavior). Such programs have shown promising results. The National Survey on Drug Use and Health (2005) estimated that approximately 78% of 12- to 17-year-old students had heard or seen drug or alcohol prevention messages during the previous year. The survey also noted that alcohol, cigarette, and illicit drug use were lower for students who were exposed to such messages in school.

Appropriately designed and implemented school-based prevention programs can prevent or reduce negative behaviors; however, accumulating research indicates that negative behaviors do not exist in isolation, so programs that address multiple co-occurring negative behaviors are likely to be of greater benefit. An example of this type of program is the Positive Action program, a comprehensive K–12 social and emotional development program that has demonstrated substantial effects on reducing multiple problem behaviors (substance abuse, violent behavior, and sexual activity; Beets et al., 2009). Occupational therapy practitioners should become familiar with and help support the prevention programs offered in their school districts and communities in order to encourage participation and reinforce the knowledge and skills gained from participation. Information related to bullying and friendship issues can be found in Appendix D.

Summaries of Evidence From Systematic Reviews of Universal Services

Universal Social Skills Programs

The first theme within Tier 1 focuses on programs related to social skills. There were 18 studies in this theme, with subthemes of social–emotional learning, social skills training, cognitive strategies, incorporating stories, parent education, and conflict resolution and bullying prevention.

One Level I meta-analysis (Durlak, Weissberg, Dymnicki, Taylor, & Schellinger, 2011) evaluated the effectiveness of universal whole school SEL programs and found that, compared to controls, participants in the intervention group demonstrated significantly improved social and emotional skills. The authors also found improved behavior, academic performance, and attitudes following participation in SEL programs.

Another Level I meta-analysis (Wells, Barlow, & Stewart-Brown, 2003) evaluated the effectiveness of universal approaches for mental health promotion and disease prevention. Programs that adopted a whole-school approach, that were implemented continuously for more than a year, and that focused on the promotion of mental health as opposed to the prevention of mental illness were successful. A Level I randomized controlled trial (RCT) that evaluated a social–emotional curriculum to prevent conduct disorders with students in Grades 1 through 3 found no difference in social competence at a 3-year follow-up (Conduct Problems Prevention Research Group, 2002). However, children in the intervention group were less likely to exhibit serious conduct problems compared to children in the control group.

Two studies examined social skills programs. Durlak, Weissberg, and Pachan (2010), in a Level I meta-analysis, evaluated the effectiveness of after-school programs that incorporated a goal of either social skills or other personal skills. Participants in after-school programs had improvements in social behaviors, bonding to school, and reduction in problem behaviors. Similar results were found in a Level III study conducted by DeMar (1997) that examined the effectiveness of social skills programming for children in at-risk families.

There were mixed results from four Level I studies (Kraag, Zeegers, Kok, Hosman, & Abu-Saad, 2006 [meta-analysis]; Mulcahy & Schachter, 1982 [randomized control group]; Tuttle, Campbell-Heider, & David, 2006 [RCT]; Vaughn & Ridley, 1983 [RCT]) that addressed various subthemes. Kraag and colleagues (2006) found improved coping skills for interventions that included problem-solving training, and Vaughn and Ridley (1983) found improved peer interaction for preschoolers for an intervention that included problem-solving training. Mulcahy and Schachter (1982) found no difference when they compared cognitive self-modeling and counseling for adolescents, and Tuttle and colleagues (2006) found no difference between cognitive skills training and a group health outreach program to reduce risk behaviors in adolescents.

The impact of parent education on children's behaviors was studied in two Level I RCTs. Wahler and Meginnis (1997) found that education in the use of mirroring or praise in parents of elementary school children resulted in higher child compliance and higher satisfaction between child and mother compared to controls. Walker and colleagues (1998) examined the effectiveness of a multi-component universal program, including parent instruction, to prevent school antisocial behaviors in at-risk kindergarteners. Those in the intervention group were reported to have less aggressive behavior at follow-up than those in the control group.

Five studies examined the effectiveness of school-based universal programs to prevent bullying and violence. Vreeman and Carroll (2007) reported inconclusive evidence for bullying prevention programs in a Level I systematic review. In a more recent systematic review and meta-analysis, Ttofi and Farrington (2009) reported that school-based anti-bullying programs were effective in reducing bullying and victimization by approximately 20% compared to controls. The authors reported that the most important components of an anti-bullying program were parent education, improved playground supervision, and classroom management.

Lefebvre-Pinard and Reid (1980 [Level I RCT]) found that social conflict training and modeling had positive effects on communication, and Stevahn, Johnson, Johnson, Oberle, and Wahl (2000 [Level I RCT]) reported that students assigned to an intervention of daily conflict resolution training had increased knowledge of negotiation procedures compared to controls. A Level III before–after study (Bosworth, Espelage, & DuBay, 1998) evaluated the effectiveness of a computer-based violence prevention program and found that adolescent participants had improved conflict management skills and prosocial behaviors.

Universal Health Promotion Programs

The second theme within Tier 1 included universal programs related to health promotion. Subthemes identified within health promotion were stress management, health literacy, back education, and yoga.

A Level I meta-analysis (Kraag et al., 2006) evaluated the effectiveness of school-based stress management and coping skills programs for children in grades 3 through 8. Nineteen studies were included in the meta-analysis, and the results indicated that although there were positive effects for reducing stress and improving coping skills for study participants, there was no effect for self-efficacy.

One Level I RCT (Pinto-Foltz, Logsdon, & Myers, 2011) evaluated the effectiveness of a mental health literacy program for adolescents. Although there was no difference in mental health literacy as measured by knowledge or attitudes about mental illness between intervention and control groups at a 1-week follow-up, mental health literacy did improve at 4 and 8 weeks for those in the intervention group.

Studies of the effectiveness of back injury prevention education programs were reported in two studies (Cardon, De Clercq, & DeBourdeaudhuij, 2002 [Level II]; Geldhof, Cardon, DeBourdeaudhuij, & De Clercq, 2007 [Level I]) with follow-up periods at 1 year and 2 years. At the 1-year follow-up, the results indicated that health promotion programs targeting back education were effective in reducing back and neck pain for elementary school children (Cardon et al., 2002). At the 2-year follow-up, more children in the back education group reported using favorable biomechanical back posture principles when lifting objects, wearing backpacks, and sitting, compared to controls.

Three studies examined the effect of yoga and yoga-based interventions on health promotion for children and adolescents. One Level I systematic review (Galantino, Galbavy, & Quinn, 2008) evaluated 10 studies and reported that yoga was effective in improving cardiorespiratory function,

grip strength, flexibility, and body composition. The results of studies of neuromuscular function are inconclusive. An additional Level I systematic review (Birdee et al., 2009) evaluated 26 studies in a variety of populations from 0 to 21 years. The results indicated that there is preliminary evidence that yoga is beneficial for physical fitness and cardiorespiratory health in children and adolescents. A Level II nonrandomized controlled trial of 62 fourth- and fifth-grade inner city students participating in an after-school yoga program (Berger, Silver, & Stein, 2009) found that those in the yoga group reported using negative behaviors less in response to stress compared to those in the control group. There were no differences between groups for global self-worth and perceptions of physical well-being.

A Level I meta-analysis (Waters et al., 2011) provided strong evidence that childhood obesity programs affect body mass index, in particular for children ages 6 through 12 years. Promising strategies for occupational therapy practitioners include the following: developing a school curriculum that includes healthy eating and physical activity, increasing physical activity and movement skills during school, providing environments and cultural practices to support healthy eating and increased physical activity, and providing support to teachers and parents to increase healthy eating and physical activity.

Universal Play/Recreation/Leisure Programs

The third theme in Tier 1 is interventions related to play, recreation, or leisure. Subthemes were recreational programs focusing on individual interests of participants, structured arts programs primarily using drama, and recreational activity programs that stressed cooperation and team building.

A Level I RCT (McNeil, Wilson, Siever, Ronca, & Mah, 2009) studied the use of recreation facilitators or connectors in after-school programs in Alberta, Canada, for Grades 3 through 5 in areas of high unemployment. The recreation facilitators worked with children and families to increase involvement in recreational activities. Although students in the intervention group increased their participation in physical activity compared to those in the control group, there were no differences between groups on a skill-based activity subscale. A Level II nonrandomized study (Jones & Offord, 1989) compared skill-based recreational programs for children ages 5 through 15 years in a variety of areas to traditional recreation programs without skill-based training. Children in the skill-based group increased their proficiency in activities such as hockey, dance, and guitar and had some integration into community activities as compared to controls. Although there were no differences between groups on behavioral measures, there were significantly fewer follow-up police charges made against students in the intervention group.

Three studies examined the impact of involvement in performing arts activities on children and adolescents. A Level I systematic review (Daykin et al., 2008) of performing arts interventions (primarily drama) found the strongest positive outcomes were peer interaction and social skills. Two Level II nonrandomized controlled trials (Walsh-Bowers & Basso, 1999; Wright et al., 2006) found similar improvements in social skills following participation in drama programs. Wright and colleagues (2006) additionally found a significant reduction in emotional problems in the structured arts intervention in the low-income population studies compared to the controls.

Skills necessary for participation in groups and activities were explored in three studies. One Level I randomized controlled study (Kutnick & Brees, 1982) incorporated techniques for cooperation in play activities of elementary school children and found increased cooperative and decreased competitive behaviors in the intervention group. Ebbeck and Gibbons (1998 [Level I RCT]) found an improvement in self-concept following team-building activities incorporated into physical

challenges in physical education. No difference in self-esteem and the ability to work with others were seen in a Level II nonrandomized controlled study that examined the effectiveness of a bike repair program for low-income youth (Kinnevy, Healy, Pollio, & North, 1999).

Summary: Universal Services

Occupational therapy practitioners are well equipped to be active participants in the provision of universal mental health services. Attention to barriers to and opportunities for providing services to promote mental health and prevent risk factors is key to shifting from an emphasis on intervention for children already identified as having mental health and/or behavior disorders to intervention for all children. The evidence-based review just presented provides strong support for the use of social skills programming at the universal level to improve social–emotional functioning and reduce problem behaviors.

In addition, there is moderate to strong evidence to support the use of play, recreation, or leisure programming to enhance social skills and peer interaction. Programs focusing on health promotion (e.g., stress management, health literacy, back education, yoga) also have shown a range of positive outcomes, including improved social and/or physical functioning and reduced symptoms. Although not inclusive, Table 3 provides further examples of occupational therapy services at the universal level emphasizing knowledge, evaluation, and intervention.

Tier 2: Targeted Mental Health Services

Targeted interventions are designed to support children and youth who have learning, emotional, or life experiences that place them at risk of engaging in problematic behavior and/or developing mental health challenges. For example, children with physical or developmental disabilities might

Table 3. Examples of Universal (Tier 1) Occupational Therapy Services

Universal Services	School

Target: All children with and without disabilities
 	
Occupational Therapy Services
Efforts focus on:
• Creating positive environments
• Embedding whole-school SEL programming (Durlak et al., 2011)
• Promoting MH literacy
• Collaboration with caregivers, youth, and teams to promote MH awareness (e.g., serve on committees related to promoting positive MH)
• Observation of affect and participation patterns in all children
• Promote successful and enjoyable participation in occupational performance areas, including structured leisure pursuits in after-school programs (Durlak et al., 2010)
	Gain Knowledge
	• *Become knowledgeable* about state-of-the-art mental health promotion and prevention programs using reputable technical assistance centers (e.g., CASEL) and current literature.
	• *Learn about public policy* affecting children's mental health at the local, state, and national levels.
	
	Evaluation
	• *Identify* school efforts to promote mental health literacy, SEL, and the use of PBS. Support implementation in a variety of contexts (classroom, hallways, lunchroom, playground, and restrooms).
	• *Become aware* of school prevention programs focusing on risk reduction (e.g., teen pregnancy, drug use, suicide, bullying), encourage participation, and reinforce message.
	• *Evaluate lunch and recess* for factors that may impede social participation for any student.
	• *Informally observe all children* for behaviors that might suggest mental health concerns or limitations in social–emotional development. Bring concerns to the educational team.
	
	Intervention
	• *Contribute to whole school SEL programs* by embedding strategies in intervention (Durlak et al., 2011).
	• *Contribute to whole-school bully prevention programs* by embedding strategies in intervention (Ttofi & Farrington, 2009).
	• *Promote mental health literacy* efforts offered in the school. Collaborate with health educators and school nurses to promote schoolwide mental health literacy activities (Pinto-Foltz et al., 2011).
	• *Promote mental and physical health promotion* by embedding stress management and coping skills (Kraag et al, 2006); *yoga* (Berger et al., 2009; Birdee et al., 2009).
	• *Provide in-service education* to teachers and staff on the following topics:
	  • *Sensory processing:* How to adapt classroom practices based on students' varying sensory needs to enhance attending and behavior regulation (e.g., The *Alert Program*).
	  • *SEL:* How to embed SEL activities within classroom routines and activities (e.g., identifying feelings, thinking about how feelings influence behavior, perspective taking; Walker, et al., 1998).
	  • Positive mental health and the type of activity participation that helps foster it.
	• *Consult* with teachers to help them recognize the student's most effective learning styles. Ensure that students are able to meet classroom demands and create modifications if needed.
	• *Clearly articulate* the scope of occupational therapy practice as including social participation, social–emotional function, and mental health (all tiers).

	Community *Become Knowledgeable* • Learn about mental health literacy initiatives at the national, state, and local level. *Evaluation* • Identify community opportunities for inclusive participation in mental health literacy efforts and foster participation. *Intervention* • Embed SEL in after-school programming (Durlak et al., 2010). • Promote opportunities for all children and youth to participate in structured leisure occupations in a variety of community settings. Help children recognize the relationship between participation in meaningful leisure interests and positive mental health. Participation in performing arts activities may foster peer interaction and social skills (Daykin et al., 2008; Walsh et al., 1991; Wright et al., 2006). • Advocate for inclusive structured leisure opportunities (arts, music, theatre, sports, clubs).

Note. PBS = positive behavioral intervention and supports; CASEL = Collaborative for Academic, Social, and Emotional Learning; PBIS = positive behavioral interventions and supports; SEL = social and emotional learning; MH = mental health.

From "Occupational Therapy Process: A Public Health Approach to Promoting Mental Health in Children and Youth" by S. Bazyk, in *Mental Health Promotion, Prevention, and Intervention With Children and Youth: A Guiding Framework for Occupational Therapy* (p. 30), by S. Bazyk (Ed.), 2011b, Bethesda, MD: AOTA Press. Copyright © 2011 by the American Occupational Therapy Association. Adapted with permission.

struggle with low self-esteem, issues related to "feeling different," or the stress associated with frequent hospitalizations. Children living in poverty are at risk of participating in risky street activities or experiencing chronic anxiety as a result of living in stressful home and neighborhood environments. Compared to universal services, the *person-occupation–environment transaction* focuses more specifically on the groups of children and youth at risk of developing mental health problems. In addition to receiving targeted services, children and youth at risk of mental health challenges also should receive and benefit from the universal services at Tier 1.

At this level (i.e., Tier 2), children generally are not identified as having a mental or emotional disorder but often begin to display subtle changes in performance. Services emphasize both prevention of mental illness and the promotion of competencies to offset early symptoms (e.g., time management, relaxation strategies). Occupational therapy practitioners may focus on adapting activities and environments to foster successful participation as well as on applying strategies to minimize early symptoms and promote positive psychological functioning (e.g., breaking down school assignments and assigning one part at a time to minimize anxiety, teaching relaxation strategies).

PBS at this level is designed to support students who have learning, behavior, or life experiences that place them at risk of engaging in problematic behavior (Freeman et al., 2006). Implementation at this level begins with a short functional behavioral assessment followed by the development of a support plan that may "include such interventions as teaching the student a functionally equivalent replacement behavior for the problem behavior or rearranging the environment to reduce the probability of the problem behavior occurring" (Kutash et al., 2006, p. 30). Students with similar needs may be provided an intervention program designed to support a small group of students and thus promote the efficient use of resources and time. An example

includes participation in a social skills group in which specific behaviors are taught, modeled, and used by the group members (Kutash et al., 2006). At this level, occupational therapists can collaborate with teachers, speech–language pathologists, or social workers to develop and cofacilitate such targeted interventions.

Evaluation

To address the needs of youth at risk of developing mental illness, it is important for occupational therapy practitioners to learn about the specific needs of this population. Although strategies to prevent problem behaviors have received significant attention in school settings, the prevention of mental illness through early identification and intervention has not. Forness (2003) suggested that applying the concept of *developmental psychopathology* can assist families and professionals in being more proactive in the early detection of emotional or behavioral disorders. Developmental psychopathology presumes that the trajectory of such disorders results from a variety of early genetic and/or environmental factors that often are overlooked (Forness, Kavale, MacMillan, Asarnow, & Duncan, 1996).

Parents, teachers, and related-services providers who interact with youth daily may become aware of and concerned about early symptoms and/or mild functional impairments but may not recognize them as *prodromal*—early symptoms of a psychiatric disorder. Inherent in the concept of developmental psychopathology is the need for early detection and primary prevention—of "frontloading" efforts at the earliest signs of trouble instead of "backloading" efforts long after a diagnosis is confirmed (Forness, 2003).

Retrospective studies have indicated that children with prodromal signs of emotional disorders are often misidentified as having a learning disability or related problems in schools (Lopez, Forness, MacMillan, Bocian, & Gresham, 1996). Certain special education designations, such as a learning disability or speech/language problems, tend to serve as the gatekeeping categories of first resort for students with mental health problems (Hoagwood & Johnson, 2003). In addition, researchers found that whereas eligibility for special education occurred at a mean age of 7.8 years, parents reported recognizing that something was wrong at 3.5 years (Duncan, Forness, & Harsough, 1995).

Although the functional analysis of behavior and positive behavioral supports have been widely applied in schools to address behavior, attention to early detection of prodromal signs of a possible psychiatric disorder has been lacking (Forness, 2003). Universal and targeted services ought to include systematic attention to interdisciplinary screening and referral for mental health disorders. Occupational therapists, with their background in psychopathology and behavior, can play an important role in such early detection, screening, and intervention.

Children with and without physical or emotional disabilities are likely, at some point in their lives, to struggle with situational stressors such as parental divorce, the death of a family member, living in poverty, friendship issues, bullying, or academic challenges. During such times, character strengths, coping strategies, and environmental supports can serve as important buffers in preventing mental ill health (Catalano et al., 2002). While interacting with and observing children, occupational therapy practitioners can make a habit of tuning in to possible situational stressors and advocating for and developing services to counteract stressors and build competencies (e.g., bereavement support groups, participation in after-school clubs).

Evaluation efforts at this level need to emphasize efficient but careful screening for subtle changes in behavior and functional skills. Within school settings, students are not identified as needing special education at this level and, as such, will not be officially included in the therapist's caseload. Specifically, some children with mild mental disorders display symptoms that are not immediately apparent and thus often go undetected (Koppelman, 2004). For example, a child who is mildly depressed might be quiet and withdrawn and underperform academically, whereas a child with mild attention deficit hyperactivity disorder (ADHD) may have difficulty focusing and getting homework completed. Anxiety might cause excessive stress for the child required to speak in front of the class.

Occupational therapy practitioners can use both informal and formal evaluation strategies to identify risk, changes in behavior or functional skills, or the early presence of mental health problems in relevant occupational performance areas. Examples of selected assessments of psychosocial function are highlighted in Table 4. A variety of strategies can be used, including observations of performance and social interaction, informal interviews of the student or teacher, or screening assessments.

Because teachers' preprofessional education does not generally prepare them to recognize mental health problems, occupational therapists can play a role in early identification and *psychoeducation* (Koller & Bertel, 2006). Educating teachers about the early signs of mental illness and proactive strengths-based prevention strategies may help them become more involved in early identification of problems and the development of appropriate classroom accommodations.

Intervention

After the evaluation process, a range of early intervention activities can be implemented. At this level, occupational therapists may collaborate with teachers, social workers, or other mental health providers to develop and cofacilitate such selective interventions. The number of children with subthreshold mental health issues remains unidentified; thus, early intervention and prevention is needed before problems escalate (Koller & Bertel, 2006).

Table 4. Evaluation at the Targeted and Intensive Levels: Selected Assessments Focusing on Social Participation, Occupational Performance, and Quality of Life in Children and Youth

Assessment	Purpose
Assessment Scale for Positive Character Traits for Developmental Disabilities (ASPeCT–DD) (Woodard, 2009)	Designed to measure the presence and strength of selected strengths-based traits in persons with developmental disabilities considered to be associated with level of happiness and/or quality of life.
CAPE/PAC: Children's Assessment of Participation and Enjoyment (CAPE) and Preferences for Activities of Children (PAC) (King et al., 2004)	Focus is on assessment of participation or engagement in activities—recreational, physical, and social.
Child Health Questionnaire (CHQ) (Waters, Salmon, & Wake, 2000)	Designed to measure functional health status, well-being, and health outcomes of children age 0 to 18 years. Measures 12 domains of health such as behavior, bodily pain, general health, and mental health.
Devereux Student Strengths Assessment (K–8) (DESSA) (LeBuffe, Shapiro, & Naglieri, 2009) Devereux Early Childhood Assessment for Infants and Toddlers (DECA–I/T) Devereux Early Childhood Assessment for Preschoolers (DECA)	Strengths-based assessments grounded in resiliency theory to measure social–emotional competency and school success. A useful assessment to measure changes as a result of social and emotional learning (SEL) programming.
ITSEA/BITSEA Comprehensive Kit **ITSEA (Infant–Toddler Social–Emotional Assessment)** **BITSEA (Brief Infant–Toddler Social–Emotional Assessment)** (Briggs-Gowan & Carter, 2006)	ITSEA—Screen for social–emotional problems. BITSEA—In-depth analysis of emerging social–emotional development and intervention guidance; 17 subscales in 4 domains; Parent Form and Child Care Provider Form.
OT PAL (Occupational Therapy Psychosocial Assessment of Learning) (Townsend et al., 1999)	Assesses the psychosocial aspects of a student's performance within the classroom as a part of the evaluation to determine student–environment fit.
PEGS: Perceived Efficacy and Goal Setting System (Missiuna, Pollock, & Law, 2004)	An innovative and motivating tool that enables young children to reflect on their strengths and abilities and identify areas of daily challenge. The collaborative goal setting involves children and their families in identifying priorities for intervention.
School Function Assessment (SFA) (Coster, Deeney, Haltwanger, & Haley, 1998)	Designed to measure student's performance in functional tasks that support *participation in academic and social aspects* of elementary school. *Focus* is on *nonacademic* aspects of school function that support mastery in academics.
Social Skills Rating System (SSRS) (Gresham & Elliott, 1990)	Screen and classify children suspected of having social behavior problems with three rating forms: student, teacher, and parent. Assesses social skills, problem behaviors, and academic competence.
School Setting Interview (SSI) Elementary and high school (Hoffman, Hemmingsson, & Kielhofner, 2000)	Client-centered semi-structured interview to assess student–environment fit and identify need for accommodations in physical or social contexts.
Youth Quality of Life Instrument–Research Version (YQOL–R) Seattle Quality of Life Group, University of Washington (Topolski et al., 2001)	An easy-to-understand self-administered questionnaire assessing quality of life in youth ages 11–18, including those with and without disabilities.

Note. From "Occupational Therapy Process: A Public Health Approach to Promoting Mental Health in Children and Youth" by S. Bazyk, in *Mental Health Promotion, Prevention, and Intervention With Children and Youth: A Guiding Framework for Occupational Therapy* (p. 37), by S. Bazyk (Ed.), 2011b, Bethesda, MD: AOTA Press. Copyright © 2011 by the American Occupational Therapy Association. Adapted with permission.

Interventions at this level include a combination of modifications to the environment, modification of the task, and/or enhanced opportunities to engage in health-promoting occupations. An example of modification to the environment is providing color-coded notebooks for a child with ADHD and encouraging teachers to embed movement breaks for the same child. Modification of the task might involve reducing expectations for a child demonstrating anxiety by breaking down a homework assignment and giving one segment at a time. Enhanced opportunities to engage in health-promoting occupations could involve participation in an activity-based grief support group for children experiencing the loss of a family member or friend.

Occupation-Based Groups

Although intervention might involve consultation with the teacher, child, and/or family, the use of occupation-based group interventions are particularly appropriate at the targeted level. "In these groups, children develop skills, productive habits, and performance patterns that will support their ability to successfully cope with the social and task demands in their daily occupations" (Olson, 2011, p. 98). Occupational therapy has had a long tradition of using groups as an important context for intervention.

In addition to participation in meaningful occupation, occupation-based groups are designed to foster peer interaction, group process, and leader involvement aimed at fostering change at an individual and group level (Schwartzberg, 2003). Purposeful activities, such as arts and crafts, games, or cooking activities, are used to enhance skill development in various occupations and improve interpersonal and intrapersonal learning (Bruce & Borg, 1993). During the activity, the occupational therapy practitioner fosters group process and the development of social–emotional competencies (e.g., social skills, identification and expression of feelings, a positive group identity).

Group process is enhanced by considering the following five factors when planning, running, and reviewing the group: (1) maximum involvement through group-centered action, (2) a maximum sense of individual and group identity, (3) a "flow" experience, (4) spontaneous involvement of members, and (5) member support and feedback (Schwartzberg, 2003). Occupational therapists receive training in group dynamics and group facilitation.

Research suggests that children who demonstrate personal or social difficulties benefit more from small groups that provide a supportive environment and an opportunity to develop positive relationships with caring adults than those who receive individual interventions (Blum & Rinehart, 1997). In addition, small therapy groups have been found to be as effective as individual therapy (Shechtman & Ben-David, 1999).

The focus of targeted interventions will vary depending on the specific issues faced by the at-risk group; these are outlined in Table 5.

School Settings

General education students demonstrating behavioral or learning difficulties because of mental health challenges may be provided "coordinated early intervening services" even if special education or related services are not needed according to the 2004 amendments to IDEA (§ 613(f)). Another way in which services may be offered for students who do not qualify for special education is through Section 504 of the Rehabilitation Act of 1973. For many students with mild mental disorders, accommodations that are provided under Section 504 are sufficient for enhancing school functioning.

Small group interventions also may be developed jointly by occupational therapists and other team members to serve students with similar needs (Freeman et al., 2006). SEL groups might be cofacilitated by an occupational therapist and speech–language pathologist for students with Asperger syndrome, for example. Occupation-based SEL

Table 5. Targeted Occupational Therapy Services for At-Risk Children and Youth

At-Risk Condition	Associated Mental Health Risks	Occupational Performance Risks	Suggested Occupational Therapy Interventions
Physical disabilities (Petrenchik, King, & Batorowicz, 2011)	• Overemphasis on rehabilitation of physical impairments overshadows attention to social and emotional needs • More likely than typical peers to encounter negative social environments (stigmatized, marginalized, socially excluded, and bullied) • ~1 in 3 children with developmental disabilities are identified as having a co-occurring mental health condition such as anxiety and depression (Schwartz, Garland, Waddell, & Harrison, 2006)	• May have fewer opportunities to participate in extracurricular activities, resulting in boredom and delayed skill development • Social isolation may result in delayed social skills, lack of friends, and limited opportunities to develop extracurricular interests • Poor self-confidence, depression, and/or anxiety may contribute further to social isolation	• Promote a balanced view of health, including attention to both physical and emotional needs of the child. • Foster sustained participation in enjoyable neighborhood- and community-based out-of-school activities to promote the development of interests and friends and to build on strengths and talents. Such positive experiences help buffer the effects of life adversities and promote positive mental health. • Encourage the child to express and process feelings related to reduced physical functioning. • Help create school and community environments that are inclusive, stimulating, satisfying, and enjoyable. • Contribute to whole-school approaches emphasizing disability awareness and acceptance of differences.
ADHD, LD, DCD (Poulsen, 2011; Young, 2007)	• Low self-esteem due to difficulties in school and home performance • Social exclusion • Anxiety • Depression	• *School.* Failure to attend to details, careless errors, avoids challenging academic tasks that require sustained mental effort, frequent shifts in attention, may have visual perception or reading problems (LD), difficulty organizing school materials in locker or desk, forgets homework • *ADLs.* Messy eating or drinking; irregular sleeping • *IADLs.* Disorganized bedroom and study space, homework incomplete, poor follow-through with chores • *Leisure.* Inattention to instructions, performance erratic, difficulty waiting turn, may have coordination problems (DCD) • *Social participation.* May be teased or bullied for poor performance	• Encourage the identification and expression of feelings by applying SEL strategies. • Help children explore and successfully participate in extracurricular leisure interests based on areas of strength to enhance feelings of competence and autonomy. Provide leisure coaching if necessary (Ziviani et al., 2009). • Analyze the student's sensory needs and develop a sensory diet to successful function in home, community, and school context. • Consult with teachers to modify classroom expectations and assignments based on the specific sensory and behavioral needs of the child (e.g., breaking down assignments into manageable pieces, taking tests in a distraction-free area). These accommodations may take the form of a 504 Plan. • Help parents and teachers understand the reasons for the child's behaviors and offer support and solutions for changing and adapting the unwanted behaviors. • Modify the environment and tasks to foster organization and the development of routines (e.g., using color coding).

(Continued)

Table 5. Targeted Occupational Therapy Services for At-Risk Children and Youth *(Cont.)*

At-Risk Condition	Associated Mental Health Risks	Occupational Performance Risks	Suggested Occupational Therapy Interventions
Obesity (~11% U.S. population) **Overweight** (~25%) Children at greatest risk of obesity are those living in poverty or having a disability (Bazyk, 2011c)	• Poor self-esteem and body image • Anxiety • Depression • May experience the negative effects associated with weight bias • Eating disorders (binge dieting and eating)	• *Social participation challenges.* Difficulty making and keeping friends due to weight bias • Higher risk of being bullied • Sleep/rest challenges due to risk of sleep apnea • *Limited play/leisure.* May find physical activities too challenging	• Emphasize "health at any size" versus weight loss. • Teach children about healthy food choices. • Work with school officials to decrease the availability of foods high in fat and sugar in the cafeteria and in vending machines. • Develop after-school programs that foster participation in enjoyable physical activities and healthy cooking. • Consult with school personnel to develop enjoyable physical activities during recess. • Work with school official to prevent weight-biased bullying. • Embed SEL strategies to help children identify feelings and develop positive coping strategies.
Grieving loss The conflicted feelings caused by change due to loss; *Examples:* death of parent, friend, or pet; parental divorce, moving to a new home (Bazyk, 2011c)	• Stress associated with loss may result in a range of behavioral changes (emotional withdrawal, regressive behaviors) • Anxiety • Depression • Difficulty concentrating at school • Psychosomatic complaints (headaches, stomachaches)	• ADL changes (altered eating patterns, bedwetting) • Altered sleep and rest, including excessive or limited sleep • Difficulty concentrating in school; drop in grades • Social withdrawal and friendship issues • Loss of interest in play/leisure activities	• Create a grief support team that meets 4 times per year to review bereavement literature and develop procedures for helping students return to school following a loss. • Teach children how to provide support to friends who are grieving. • Help teachers recognize emotional and behavioral changes associated with grieving and suggest strategies for modifying expectations and providing support. • Encourage participation in enjoyable but low-stress activities with close friends to minimize feelings of isolation. • Use creative arts occupations to help children express feelings of loss either in small group or individual sessions (e.g., journaling, making memory boards, scrapbooking) • Mention the person who died in everyday conversation to encourage the student to talk about what he or she valued in the relationship. • Be aware of "grief triggers" such as birthdays and holidays. Reassure children that heightened emotions during these times are a natural part of grieving.

(Continued)

Table 5. Targeted Occupational Therapy Services for At-Risk Children and Youth *(Cont.)*

At-Risk Condition	Associated Mental Health Risks	Occupational Performance Risks	Suggested Occupational Therapy Interventions
Poverty (~16% U.S. population) **Low income** (~37%) (Bazyk, 2011c)	• Depression • Anxiety • Substance abuse • Aggressive behavior	• Sleep problems due to stressful environment • Obesity due to limited access to fresh fruits, vegetables, and safe playgrounds • Limited opportunities to engage in extracurricular leisure activities resulting in boredom and participation in risky behavior	• Help parents consciously steer children away from street influences by monitoring free time and friendships. • Promote engagement in structured leisure activities outside of school such as sports, church groups, and creative arts in positive environments • Foster SEL—identifying feelings and reflecting on how feelings influence behavior.
Children who have experienced trauma • Community, school, and domestic violence • Physical abuse, sexual abuse, and neglect • Separation from parents • Natural disasters • Medical trauma (Bloom, 1995; Stein et al., 2003)	• PTSD • ADHD • Anxiety • Depression • Communication disorder • Conduct disorder • Eating disorders • Oppositional defiant disorder • May engage in self-destructive and risky behaviors	• Sleep disorders • *ADL.* May demonstrate poor hygiene and self-care • *Social participation.* Social withdrawal and isolation; may have difficulty trusting people • *School.* Poor attendance, low grades, difficulty concentrating, and behavioral challenges • *Play/leisure.* Loss of interest in leisure activities and play	• Modify home and school environments to create safe, secure, and sensory friendly spaces (e.g., weighted lap pads, fidget toys, rocking chairs, soothing lights). • Apply the Sanctuary Model to help create collaborative and healing environments that promote recovery from trauma (www.santuaryweb.com). • Structure predictable routines in home and school. • Tune into the child's affect and emotional responses, and triggers to problem behaviors. Develop strategies to modify them. • Offer small occupation-based groups to provide opportunities to share feelings, learn new coping strategies, and engage in enjoyable creative occupations. • Provide leisure coaching to help children identify and participate in enjoyable extracurricular activities. • Teach relaxation skills including yoga, deep breathing, and progressive relaxation.

(Continued)

groups also can be offered to other at-risk groups, including low-income urban youth (Bazyk, 2005; Bazyk & Bazyk, 2009).

Home and Community

In addition to addressing school function, attention to home and community participation is essential. Close collaboration with caregivers regarding early intervention and carryover into the home needs to be ongoing. In particular, the promotion of successful participation in social and structured leisure activities during out-of-school time is important for building competencies and offering enjoyable experiences that promote a sense of emotional well-being.

Approaches for fostering participation in meaningful community-based occupations have

Table 5. Targeted Occupational Therapy Services for At-Risk Children and Youth *(Cont.)*

At-Risk Condition	Associated Mental Health Risks	Occupational Performance Risks	Suggested Occupational Therapy Interventions
Children at risk of psychosis and demonstrating signs of prodromal phase • Subtle, experiential symptoms may ebb and flow in frequency and intensity up to 4 years before the onset of an illness (Downing, 2011)	• Cognitive changes in functioning such as difficulty concentrating or remembering information; may experience jumbled thoughts or confusion • May experience perceptual distortions such as hearing one's name called or increased sensitivity to sounds • May demonstrate behavioral changes such as withdrawal or increased irritability • May become suspicious of others and/or fearful for no reason • May demonstrate jumbled speech or writing	• *Social participation.* Deteriorating social function altering relationships with family and friends; may become socially isolated • *School.* Problems staying focused in class or during studies and may demonstrate a drop in grades • *Work.* May demonstrate declining performance such as tardiness and a failure to complete work assignments • *Leisure.* May drop out of extracurricular activities • *ADLs.* May demonstrate dramatic changes in appetite and difficulty in dressing and/or hygiene • *Sleep/rest.* May demonstrate dramatic changes in sleep either difficulty sleeping or excessive sleep	• Offer in-services to school personnel and families about sensory preferences and how to modify the environment to decrease stress and promote positive functioning. • Offer small group sessions to foster participation in enjoyable activities to reduce stress and promote socialization. • Consult with teachers and parents to make accommodations to reduce stress and enhance participation such as decreasing activity demands; assisting with organization of a task; reducing environmental stimulation; and developing routines that include exercise, healthy nutrition, and good sleep hygiene.

Note. ADHD = attention deficit hyperactivity disorder; ADL = activities of daily living; DCD = developmental coordination disorder; IADL = instrumental activities of daily living; LD = learning disabilities; PTSD = posttraumatic stress disorder; SEL = social and emotional learning.

been proposed. For example, Engaging and Coaching for Health (EACH)–Child provides strategies for promoting sustained physical activity in children through a process of exploration and engagement, coaching, and scaffolded experiences (Ziviani, Poulsen, & Hansen, 2009). In a related way, occupational performance coaching has been proposed as an approach to help parents and their children participate more successfully in self-identified home and community occupations (Graham, Rodger, & Ziviani, 2009).

The first step in promoting participation is to communicate the many intrapersonal and interpersonal benefits of structured leisure participation to children, families, and community leaders. Special efforts to promote participation might be necessary for children at risk of limited participation due to restricted access and availability (e.g., low-income urban youth). Children and youth with developmental disabilities are also at risk of limited participation in structured leisure, which may lead to feelings of isolation, restricted social interaction, and boredom. Children who are experiencing early signs of mental illness (e.g., depression) may display little interest in or motivation to participate in extracurricular activities and may need support and encouragement to initiate such participation.

To promote participation in structured leisure, it is important to know one's community. Specifically, becoming aware of the range of activity options—including sports, arts, music, outdoor, community recreation, and club-related opportunities—is essential. Personally visiting settings and meeting directors is one strategy that would allow the occupational therapy practitioner to assess whether the context is open to youth with disabilities or mental health problems and whether the setting might support positive functioning (e.g., physical and psychological safety, appropriate structure, supportive relationships, opportunities for belonging, positive social norms, and opportunities for skill building; Eccles & Gootman, 2002). Once the occupational therapist is aware of community options, a discussion of possible interests can take place based on the child's personality, developmental stage, and ability level. Identifying activities that are meaningful, enjoyable, interesting, and that provide the "just-right" challenge is key to motivating engagement (Poulsen, Rodger, & Ziviani, 2006).

"Identifying an interest is the first step in achieving a goal; however, to engage in an activity relies on sustaining that interest through supportive environments and well-targeted instructional strategies" (Ziviani et al., 2009, p. 264). Adapting initial entry into the activity might be necessary depending on the individual's specific needs. For example, a child with anxiety might agree to participate in a new activity if given the option to bring a friend or simply observe the first session. Consulting with the instructor or coach to modify the environment, activity, or interaction to support successful participation is another strategy for ensuring sustained involvement. Being available for ongoing consultation and problem solving also are advised.

When feasible, fostering participation in integrated community settings for children with disabilities is suggested. Wehmeyer and Bolding (1999) found that individuals who lived or worked in community-based settings were more self-determined, had more choices, and were more satisfied than those living in congregate settings. See Table 5 for information on at-risk groups and suggested occupational therapy services, and see Table 6 for examples of occupational therapy services at the targeted level emphasizing evaluation and intervention at the in

school, health care, and community levels. See Boxes 4, 5, and 6 for clinical vignettes of targeted intervention for a child at risk of mental health challenges.

Summaries of Evidence From Systematic Reviews of Targeted/ Selective Services

Targeted interventions were examined in Tier 2, which included the same themes of Tier 1 of social skills, health promotion, and play/leisure/recreation. The subthemes within the social skills program are related to the populations studied. These subthemes include children and adolescents who have been rejected by peers, are at risk of behavioral problems or aggressive behaviors, have learning disabilities and/or ADHD, have intellectual impairments and/or developmental delay, or are teenage mothers.

Targeted Social Skills Interventions

Seven studies focused on activity-based social skills programs for children and adolescents who have been rejected or disliked by peers or for adolescents experiencing social difficulty (Bierman & Furman, 1984 [Level I RCT]; Bierman, Miller, & Stabb, 1987 [Level I RCT]; Csapo, 1986 [Level I RCT]; Hepler & Rose, 1988 [Level II nonrandomized controlled trial]; Jackson & Marziller, 1983 [Level I RCT]; Mevarech & Kramarksi, 1993 [Level II nonrandomized controlled trial]; Morris, Messer, & Gross, 1995 [Level I RCT]). The results of these studies indicated that social skills training improves social interaction, peer acceptance, and social standing for children and adolescents who are disliked or have been rejected by peers. The results of a study of adolescents with social difficulty (Jackson & Marziller, 1983) indicate, however, that there was no difference between a social skill intervention compared to a wait-list control condition.

Fifteen studies examined the effectiveness of social skills programming for children and adolescents who were classified as at risk, aggressive,

Table 6. Examples of Targeted (Tier 2) Occupational Therapy Services

Targeted Services Selective or targeted intervention for at-risk children and youth	School
	Obtain Knowledge
	• *Learn* about early signs of a variety of mental illnesses (e.g., depression, anxiety, obsessive–compulsive disorder, schizophrenia) and how such symptoms might manifest themselves in school and home settings
Targeted Population: Children and Youth	• *Become knowledgeable* about strategies for early intervention.
• With any disability (CP, ASD, LD, ADHD, etc.)	**Evaluation**
• Those experiencing loss (e.g., through death, divorce, military deployment)	• *Use both informal and formal evaluation strategies* to identify risk, changes in behavior or functional skills, or the early presence of mental health problems.
• Who are overweight or obese	• *Evaluate social participation* with peers during all school activities, including recess and lunch.
• Living in poverty	• *Analyze the sensory, social, and cognitive demands of school tasks* and recommend adaptations to support a student's participation.
• Demonstrating early signs of a mental health disorder (e.g., anxiety) or sudden changes in behaviors	**Intervention**
• Who struggle with friendships and/or problem behaviors	• *Develop and run activity-based social skills group programs* to foster social participation for students struggling with peer interaction and/or problem behaviors (Bierman & Furman, 1984; Bierman et al., 1987; Csapo, 1986; Hepler & Rose, 1988; Jackson & Marziller, 1983; Mevarech & Kramarksi, 1993; Morris et al., 1995).
	• *Provide social skills programming* for children and youth with ADHD and learning disabilities (Drysdale et al., 2008; Frankel et al., 1997; Lamb et al., 1997; Wiener & Harris, 1997).
Occupational Therapy Services	• *Embedded yoga and relaxation strategies* may promote positive behavior for students with behavioral challenges (Powell et al., 2008).
Efforts involve a more direct role in evaluation and service provision and focus on all universal services, plus:	• *Implement play/recreation/leisure programming* to promote social interaction and reduce behavior problems (Anderson & Allen, 1985a, 1985b; Carter & Hughes, 2005; Gencoz, 1997; Jeffree & Cheseldine, 1984; Santomier & Kopczuk, 1981).
• Screening for early identification of problems in a variety of areas, including social participation, sensory processing, play/leisure	• *Provide early intervening services* or Section 504 accommodations for students demonstrating behavioral or learning difficulties due to mild mental health disorders or psychosocial issues.
• Early intervening services to promote successful participation in school, home, and community utilizing social skills, health promotion, and play/recreation/leisure programming	• *Consult with teachers* to modify learning demands and academic routines to support a student's development of specific social–emotional skills.
	• *Provide parent education* on how to adapt family routines or activities to support children's mental health, especially with high-risk children.
	• *Provide psychoeducation in-services* to educate teachers about the early signs of mental illness and appropriate accommodations.
• Small group work	Community
• Coaching	**Obtain Knowledge**
• Consultation and collaboration	• *Become knowledgeable* about the benefits of participation in structured leisure and communicate this understanding to children/youth and families.
	Evaluation
	• *Identify community recreation centers,* dance studios, sports opportunities, clubs, and other settings that offer inclusive opportunities for participation.
	Intervention
	• *Visit community settings,* meet the program directors, and explore options for youth with mental or physical needs to participate.
	• *Develop a resource guide* of positive settings for youth to participate in structured leisure activities.

Note. CP = cerebral palsy; ASD = autism spectrum disorder; LD = learning disabilities; ADHD = attention deficit hyperactivity disorder. From "Occupational Therapy Process: A Public Health Approach to Promoting Mental Health in Children and Youth" by S. Bazyk, in *Mental Health Promotion, Prevention, and Intervention With Children and Youth: A Guiding Framework for Occupational Therapy* (p. 35), by S. Bazyk (Ed.), 2011b, Bethesda, MD: AOTA Press. Copyright © 2011 by the American Occupational Therapy Association. Adapted with permission.

or antisocial (Charlebois, Normandeau, Vitaro, & Berneche, 1999 [Level III before–after study]; Conduct Problems Prevention Research Group [Level I RCT], 2002; Dubow, Huesmann, & Eron, 1987 [Level II nonrandomized controlled trial]; Kamps, Tankersley, & Ellis, 2000 [Level I RCT]; Kazdin, Bass, Siegel, & Thomas, 1989 [Level I RCT]; Lochman & Wells, 2002 [Level I RCT], 2003 [Level I RCT], 2004 [Level I RCT]; McMahon, Washburn, Felix, Yakin, & Childrey, 2000 [Level III before–after study]; Moody, Childs, & Sepples, 2003 [Level III pretest–posttest study]; Ohl, Mitchell, Cassidy, & Fox, 2008 [Level II nonrandomized controlled trial]; Rickel, Eshelman, & Loigman, 1983 [Level II nonrandomized controlled trial]; Serna, Nielsen, Lambros, & Forness, 2000 [Level I RCT]; Tankersley, Kamps, Mancina, & Weidinger, 1996 [Level I RCT]; Waddell, Hua, Garland, Peters, & McEwan, 2007 [Level I systematic review]). Although the populations and interventions that were studied varied, the overall results indicated that social skills programming results in improved attention, peer interaction, and prosocial behaviors, as well as reduced aggressive, delinquent, and antisocial behaviors. The studies also reported fewer diagnoses for conduct disorders and reductions in anxiety and depression for at-risk children.

The effectiveness of social skills programming for children and adolescents with learning disabilities and ADHD was examined in four studies

(Continued on p. 48)

Box 4. Targeted Intervention for Children With Disabilities: An Integrated Creative Arts Group Program for Children With and Without Disabilities—MasterPiece Kids

In July 2004, the Cleveland Clinic Children's Hospital for Rehabilitation received a grant to develop a Creative Arts Program for children with disabilities and their typically developing peers. Based on two Level I randomized controlled trials (Duffy & Fuller, 2000; Udwin, 1983), two Level II nonrandomized controlled trials (Sparling, Walker, & Singdahlsen, 1984; Sussman, 2009), and one Level III before–after study (Lochman, Haynes, & Dobson, 1981), structured arts and drama interventions resulted in improvements in social participation.

An interdisciplinary group of professionals, including an occupational therapist, recreation therapist, teacher, and the head of volunteer services, developed a program entitled MasterPiece Kids, targeting youth ages 6–10 years and youth age 11 years or older. Sessions range from 4 to 6 weeks long and are held after school for 2 hours. Two different art experiences are offered during each weekly session. Local artists are involved in each session and represent a variety of creative expression, including music, dance, drumming, pottery, creative writing, puppetry, and baking. Children respond best to instructors who combine structure with flexibility. Participating children are happy and eager to try every new activity. It is gratifying to offer all kinds of creative arts opportunities for all children with and without disabilities.

—Susan Gara Mastromonaco, OTR/L

Note. Adapted from "Major Approaches Useful in Addressing the Mental Health Needs of Children and Youth: Minimizing Risks, Reducing Symptoms, and Buildng Competencies" by S. Bazyk and S. Brandenburger Shasby, in *Mental Health Promotion, Prevention, and Intervention With Children and Youth: A Guiding Framework for Occupational Therapy* (p. 58), by S. Bazyk (Ed.), 2011, Bethesda, MD: AOTA Press. Copyright © 2011 by the American Occupational Therapy Association. Adapted with permission. For further information, see Duffy and Fuller (2000), Lochman et al. (1981), Lowenstein (1982), Ohl et al. (2008), Sparling et al. (1984), Sussman (2009), and Udwin (1983).

Box 5. Targeted Intervention—Case Study of a Child Who Is Medically Fragile and at Risk for Developing Mental Health Challenges

Anna, age 10, was diagnosed with nemaline rod myopathy. She is considered medically fragile, is fed by gastrostomy tube, has a tracheotomy, and requires frequent suctioning and the occasional support of a ventilator. Anna does not speak and experiences significant physical limitations. She can move only her head, eyes, and two index fingers. Despite her physical challenges, she drives a wheelchair and uses an augmentative and alternative communication (AAC) system independently, which she operates by switches.

Anna's receptive-language skills are age appropriate in two languages, Slovakian and English. Her expressive-language skills in English are at the Grade 2 level. She is bright and academically competitive. Anna lives in a small house with her older brother and parents, who emigrated from Slovakia 10 years ago. Her parents speak little English.

Anna attends a Grade 4 mainstream class, where she receives the full-time support of an educational assistant. Anna attends most classes, with exception of gym. After school, she stays at home, where she watches TV or plays on the computer, which has been adapted to her physical needs. The occupational therapist has been asked to adapt the school's written tests for Anna so that she can complete them independently and to troubleshoot the computer access at home so that she can write her homework.

During the occupational therapist's school visit, the therapist notices that Anna sits at the back of the classroom and interacts only with her educational assistant. When the therapist visits Anna at home, Anna tells her that she would like to use e-mail and asks whether she could correspond with her. When the occupational therapist inquires about her friends, Anna tells the therapist that she has two friends at school who talk to her, but she has not seen them outside of the school setting. She confides that she often feels lonely and disconnected from her peers.

Although Anna is not diagnosed with a mental health disorder at this time, she is at risk due to the social isolation she is experiencing at school, home, and the community. Specific to mental health, occupational therapy for Anna involves a range of evidence-based services, including consultation and education with parents and teachers; promotion of social participation with peers; and exploration and participation in creative recreation, leisure, and arts programming. All such interventions are used to promote mental health and prevent mental ill health for children at risk.

Evaluation and Intervention Planning

Evaluation and intervention will address Anna's psychosocial well-being; social inclusion; and meaningful participation in school, at home, and in community-based out-of-school activities. The evaluation will focus on Anna's interests and her social networks and on the qualities of her environmental settings. The occupational therapist will identify participation barriers, including (1) policies, practices, attitudes, and lack of appropriate resources and supports and (2) communication-relevant barriers. The intervention will involve creating optimal environmental settings that offer choice and opportunity and support growth-enhancing experiences for Anna. The focus will be on supporting meaningful engagement and social interactions in Anna's natural environments with a variety of people, especially her peers. The goal for Anna is to promote her mental health and prevent secondary mental health problems through positive experiences of doing and belonging, which will be achieved by using multifaceted intervention strategies with a focus on enhancing participation and social inclusion in a variety of settings.

(Continued)

Box 5. Targeted Intervention—Case Study of a Child Who Is Medically Fragile and at Risk for Developing Mental Health Challenges *(Cont.)*

Participation and Inclusion at School

Anna is a competitive student; therefore, she will be supported to participate in the same activities as her peers and should be expected to meet the same educational standards. The occupational therapist's role is to assist teachers in modifying Anna's workloads; providing her with adequate time to complete tasks; and maximizing her level of physical independence, thereby allowing her to focus on the same curricular content as her peers. This intervention should focus not only on Anna's independent (and solitary) participation in curriculum through adaptations but also on optimizing her environment to support meaningful engagement in academic activities and to encourage a sense of belonging in the classroom and school community, which will be achieved by enabling and supporting social interactions with peers and school personnel in classroom settings and during informal recess interactions. Examples of specific strategies include (1) providing structured ongoing opportunities for peer interactions, such as group projects; (2) supporting Anna's inclusion in school trips and gym class, which are fun activities offering natural opportunities for peer interaction; and (3) creating social environments that support the successful fulfillment of these opportunities (e.g., teaching school personnel and peers about communicating using AAC strategies or use of peer instruction and support by forming collaborative learning groups). Studies examining the effectiveness of social and life skills programming for children with intellectual impairments and developmental delay (Antia & Kreimeyer, 1996; Carter & Hughes, 2005; Girolametto, 1988; Kingsnorth, Healy, & MacArthur, 2007; O'Connor et al., 2007; Wade, Carey, & Wolfe, 2006) indicate that such programming improves social interaction (e.g., initiation of social interaction, conversational turn-taking), performance of life skills, and self-management.

Participation and Inclusion in Community-Based After-School Activities

During her occupational therapy assessment, Anna identifies the following interests: going to the library, dancing, participating in dramatic arts, and going for walks in the neighborhood. The occupational therapist's role is to offer choices, create opportunities, and provide supports, both directly and by serving as an intermediary and advocate. Offering choices involves inviting Anna to identify and select specific community-based programs of interest to her. Creating opportunities involves supporting Anna and her family in their advocacy efforts with community organizations and agencies such as the local library, children's theater, and dance studios to support Anna's participation in programs offered to all children. Providing supports directly and as an intermediary involves coordinating organizational and social supports, collaborating with community partners and the family to enable Anna's meaningful participation, and creating a community of informed and sensitive peers. Participation in programs of Anna's choosing will provide her with opportunities to meet peers and to gain group membership. Participation in recreation and leisure has been shown to improve social interaction in children and youth with disabilities (Anderson & Allen, 1985a, 1985b; Carter & Hughes, 2005; Gencoz, 1997; Jeffree & Cheseldine, 1984; Santomier & Kopczuk, 1981).

Anna also has expressed an interest in walking in her neighborhood. Anna's family will be encouraged to invite neighborhood children of Anna's age to join them for walks in the neighborhood and to create opportunities for them to visit Anna at home, providing further opportunities to build meaningful relationships. Because of her strong computing abilities, Anna can maintain her new peer relationships through social media such as e-mail, instant messaging, Facebook, and interactive online games, all of which would allow her stay connected with her peers outside of school.

(Continued)

Box 5. Targeted Intervention—Case Study of a Child Who Is Medically Fragile and at Risk for Developing Mental Health Challenges *(Cont.)*

Participation at Home

Anna expresses an interest in helping her mother with cooking. The occupational therapist will discuss with Anna and her mother the tasks that interest Anna and strategies for involving her on a regular basis. For example, Anna can read recipes aloud to her mother as she is cooking, she can become involved in cooking decisions (e.g., selecting pizza toppings or cake decorations), and she can be responsible for creating shopping lists and participating in grocery shopping. The latter will offer Anna opportunities to get out of the house, to meet and talk with people in her community, and to expand her social networks.

Participation in Special Events

Anna enjoys writing poetry, and the occupational therapist can encourage her to share her expressive work with others. For example, the occupational therapist can assist Anna in arranging a poetry reading at her school or local library or encourage her to join or form a poetry club. The therapist also can play a role in enabling Anna to publish her poems through the International Society for Augmentative and Alternative Communication (ISAAC) and to present her work at conferences for people who use AAC or health care professionals (e.g., an ISAAC conference or an Independence, Community, and Empowerment conference). Participation in such events will provide opportunities for Anna to meet others who use AAC strategies, to expand her social networks, and to develop greater confidence in herself and her creative abilities.

Models of Service Provision

In keeping with best practice principles (Dunn, 2000), the occupational therapist provides direct and indirect services in Anna's natural activity settings.

Child- and Family-Centered Interventions

Direct intervention with Anna focuses on adapting Anna's communication system so it is most effective for social interaction and participation in specific activity settings. The goal is to create effective AAC systems to provide opportunities for Anna to easily interact with people in different environments.

Collaboration with a speech–language pathologist is important to adjust the AAC system to specific emerging needs (e.g., programming new vocabulary that is setting specific, reorganize existing vocabulary for targeted efficient access). For example, Anna identifies that she would like to interact with her non–English-speaking grandmother, who will be visiting soon. Collaboration with a computer technician or vendor may be needed to add a second language to Anna's AAC system. Also, the occupational therapist can help Anna prepare an "about me" speech so she can introduce herself to new peers and instructors in community programs.

Home-based interventions with the family focus on (1) caregiving strategies for a child with complex needs; (2) balancing family needs and routines; and (3) developing strategies for supporting Anna's participation at home, at school, and in the community. In the area of participation, Anna's parents are provided with information on specific community-based opportunities available to Anna and her family. Together, the family and the occupational therapist explore and discuss the available options and develop a plan for enabling Anna's participation in a setting of her choosing. For her participation in this area to be

(Continued)

Box 5. Targeted Intervention—Case Study of a Child Who Is Medically Fragile and at Risk for Developing Mental Health Challenges *(Cont.)*

sustainable, the occupational therapist must make certain that the opportunities Anna chooses fit with the needs and resources of the entire family (e.g., time, money, transportation).

Community-Based Intervention
Community-based interventions involve accompanying Anna during her initial participation in various community programs and settings (e.g., dance studio, library, theater) to help ensure that her initial interactions with unfamiliar people are successful. Positive interaction experiences are crucial in developing positive peer relationships, and repeated unsuccessful interaction experiences produce negative peer attitudes and low motivation for future contacts.

Systems-Level Interventions
Systems-level interventions involve collaborations with and coordination among school personnel and key stakeholders from the community agencies, including administrators and instructors. The purpose is to secure services and resources for Anna; to modify policies, procedures, or practices that pose barriers to Anna's participation; and to promote the adoption of new procedures and policies that will result in sustainable participation and social inclusion. All such strategies are important for optimizing Anna's chances of achieving her full health potential. The strategies involved will include educational and consultative activities.

Educational activities include providing general education about principles of communicating using AAC and educating Anna's peers and teachers about how they can become effective communication partners, which is done through a series of structured interactive activities and by the occupational therapist's modeling of positive, respectful interactions. In these sessions with peers and school personnel, Anna serves as an educator and advocates for herself by talking about her interests, strengths, challenges, and goals. Such educational sessions are important for creating a more welcoming school climate by increasing participants' knowledge and understanding of children with disabilities. They are also important for educating others about Anna's abilities and for exploring possibilities for including Anna in school- and community-based activities. For example, the occupational therapist can help others understand how Anna can safely and successfully participate in dance using her wheelchair, thereby creating new opportunities for Anna to be involved in dance lessons and performances with her peers.

Consultations are time-limited and task-specific. Case consultations involve a series of meetings with Anna's teacher to explore ways in which the teacher can enhance Anna's participation in classroom activities and field trips. Consultations also may be provided during times of school transition, for example, when Anna changes a grade level, homeroom teacher, classroom, or school. Other areas of consultation involve a variety of community agencies and include issues of personal safety, accessibility of the built environment, and modification of tasks and the sensory environment to enable Anna's successful participation.

Note. From "Children and Youth With Disabilities: Enhancing Mental Health Through Positive Experiences of Doing and Belonging," by T. M. Petrenchik, G. A. King, & B. Batorowicz, in *Mental Health Promotion, Prevention, and Intervention With Children and Youth: A Guiding Framework for Occupational Therapy* (pp. 200–202), by S. Bazyk (Ed.), 2011, Bethesda, MD: AOTA Press. Copyright © 2011 by the American Occupational Therapy Association. Adapted with permission.

Box 6. Targeted Intervention—Case Example of a Youth at Risk of Psychosis

Allison, a 13-year-old seventh grader, is referred to the Portland Identification and Early Referral (PIER) Program by the school social worker and meets criteria for the program based on attenuated positive symptoms, a steady decline in school performance, and withdrawal from peers. She is living with her mother, stepfather, and 6-year-old half-brother. Her biological father, who carries a diagnosis of bipolar I disorder with psychosis, is not involved with her life, but her stepfather seems to be caring and involved. The school social worker is aware of the early signs of psychosis due to a recent PIER outreach training. She also is aware of Allison's biological father's history of psychosis, which places her at high risk of psychosis.

Following the research intake assessment process, the PIER occupational therapy practitioner meets with Allison and her mother for a first session. It is reported that Allison is having increasing trouble processing auditory information but does not have a learning disability. She also demonstrates a heightened response to environmental stimuli, resulting in sensory avoidance. During the Canadian Occupational Performance Measure (Law et al., 2005), Allison reports that she no longer likes school and is dissatisfied with her academic performance and socialization. She still enjoys some hobbies, such as writing poetry, which she does in her bedroom. This is an area of satisfaction for her. She tends to avoid school and is at risk of having too many absences, which could result in the need to take summer classes. Allison is not completing and/or passing in assignments, which is a performance change. In the past, she has been a conscientious student, passing in assignments on time.

Allison and her mother agree on two major goals: (1) attend school each day and (2) complete class assignments on time. They want to know what they can do to reduce stimuli so that she will be less distracted in class, feel more motivated to be social, and feel less stressed. The occupational therapy practitioner discusses the occupational therapy evaluation process and which assessment tools will provide information about Allison's cognitive and functional abilities, as well as her sensory preferences. She schedules a second assessment session for later in the week and discusses what she and Allison will do during that meeting: (1) complete the Adolescent/Adult Sensory Profile (Brown & Dunn, 2002), to better understand Allison's sensory preferences, and (2) complete the Test of Everyday Attention–Child version (Manly et al., 1998) to better understand Allison's difficulties with attention. The occupational therapy practitioner schedules a third session for Allison to participate in two activities of daily living that she chooses as part of the Assessment of Motor and Process Skills (Fisher & Bray Jones, 2010). Allison decides to make a sandwich and sweep the floor, which are two familiar activities.

Before ending the first session, the occupational therapy practitioner asks Allison and her mother to help make a plan for Allison get to school the next day. Together, they develop a detailed action plan that includes specifics about (1) how Allison will wake up (i.e., she will set her clock radio that night for earlier than usual to allow more time to get ready), (2) what will help her feel less anxious so that she will more easily leave the house (i.e., have her mother drive her to school with her best friend), and (3) whom she can contact at school if she starts to feel anxious (i.e., the school nurse, a favorite teacher). They identify specific tasks for each of them to carry out to make the plan successful. Allison and her mother create a reward system that consists of spending time together the next evening if Allison attends school on time and stays there for the day. The end result is that Allison and her mother feel more positive, hopeful, and less stressed because they have a clear plan. Mother and daughter agree to tackle the homework issue at home later that day, using some of the techniques they learn in the session with the occupational therapy practitioner.

(Continued)

Box 6. Targeted Intervention—Case Example of a Youth at Risk of Psychosis *(Cont.)*

The results of the Adolescent/Adult Sensory Profile reveal that Allison rates "much more than most people" in the areas of sensory sensitivity and sensory avoidance. This finding matches reports of Allison's recent experiences and behaviors. When she makes a sandwich and sweeps the floor for the Assessment of Motor and Process Skills activities, she demonstrates significant difficulties with executive functioning skills (especially with planning and sequencing), crossing the midline, and trunk stability. During the Test of Everyday Attention, it is clear that Allison has difficulty with divided attention, visual scanning, and verbal working memory. All of these difficulties have an impact on multiple occupational performance areas at school and home, including her desire to be social. The assessments also reveal Allison's strengths (e.g., motivation, good social skills, pleasant manner, ability to sustain attention when distractions are minimal, insight about deficits), which the occupational therapy practitioner includes in her report.

The PIER occupational therapy practitioner develops a short report that is easy for parents and school staff to understand; that is, jargon is eliminated. The report includes Allison's strengths and challenges, as well as recommendations for addressing her sensitivities, specific learning style, extracurricular leisure activities, and support for opportunities for social participation. All of the recommendations are easy to implement and nonstigmatizing, especially for the classroom setting, which is an important issue at Allison's age. The PIER occupational therapy practitioner asks the family if she can share her assessment results during the pending individual education plan meeting and if she can enlist the aid of the school occupational therapy practitioner to help implement some of the recommendations. The family agrees to both requests.

In this case example, the occupational therapy practitioner uses three approaches that have been supported in the evidence-based review for children/youth at risk for emotional and behavioral challenges— parent education, social skills interventions and supports, and extracurricular recreation/leisure activities. Working closely with parents to help them interact in positive ways with their child and effectively manage behavior is supported in the research. The impact of parent education on children's behaviors was studied in two Level I randomized controlled trials. Wahler and Meginnis (1997) found that education in the use of praise in parents of elementary school children resulted in higher child compliance and higher satisfaction between child and mother as compared to controls. Walker, Kavanagh, Stiller, Golly, Severson, and Feil (1998) examined the effectiveness of a multicomponent universal program, including parent instruction to prevent school antisocial behaviors in at-risk kindergarteners. Those in the intervention group were reported to have less–aggressive behavior at follow-up than those in the control group.

There is strong support for social skills programming for at-risk children and youth resulting in improved peer interaction and prosocial behaviors and reductions in anxiety and depression for at-risk children (Charlebois, Normandeau, Vitaro, & Berneche, 1999; Dubow, Huesmann, & Eron, 1987; Eshelman, & Loigman, 2003, 2004; Kamps, Tankersley, & Ellis, 2000; Kazdin, Bass, Siegel, & Thomas, 1989; Lochman & Wells, 2002, 2003, 2004; McMahon, Washburn, Felix, Yakin, & Childrey, 2000; Moody et al., 2003; Ohl et al., 2008; Rickel et al., 1983; Serna et al., 2000; Tankersley et al., 1996; Waddell et al., 2007). Finally, there is strong evidence to support the use of play/recreation/leisure programming to enhance social interaction and self-esteem in at-risk groups (Anderson & Allen, 1985a, 1985b; Carter & Hughes, 2005; Gencoz, 1997; Jeffree & Cheseldine, 1984; Santomier & Kopczuk, 1981).

Note. From "Occupational Therapy for Youth at Risk of Psychosis and Those With Identified Mental Illness," by D. Downing, in *Mental Health Promotion, Prevention, and Intervention With Children and Youth: A Guiding Framework for Occupational Therapy* (p. 156), by S. Bazyk (Ed.), 2011, Bethesda, MD: AOTA Press. Copyright © 2011 by the American Occupational Therapy Association. Adapted with permission.

(Continued from p. 41)
(Drysdale, Casey, & Porter-Armstrong, 2008 [Level I RCT]; Frankel, Myatt, Cantwell, & Feinberg, 1997 [Level II nonrandomized controlled trial]; Lamb, Bibby, & Wood, 1997 [Level III before–after study]; Wiener & Harris, 1997 [Level I RCT]). The results of these studies indicated that social skills training, either conducted alone or in combination with life skills programming, are effective in improving communication and social and functional skills and in reducing problem behaviors.

Seven studies examined the effectiveness of social and life skills programming for children with intellectual impairments and developmental delay (Antia & Kreimeyer, 1996 [Level II nonrandomized controlled trial]; Carter & Hughes, 2005 [Level I systematic review]; Girolametto, 1988 [Level I RCT]; Kingsnorth et al., 2007 [Level I systematic review]; O'Connor et al., 2007 [Level II nonrandomized controlled trial]; Shechtman, 2000 [Level I RCT]; Wade, Carey, & Wolfe, 2006 [Level I RCT]). The results indicated that social and life skills programming improves social interaction, particularly in the area of initiation of social interaction and conversational turn-taking. In addition, there was an improvement in performance of life skills, self-management, and compliance, and a reduction in aggression and problem behaviors.

Coren and Barlow (2001), who conducted a Level I systematic review, found that parenting programs for teenage mothers and their children resulted in improved mother–infant interaction, parental attitudes, parental knowledge, maternal mealtime communication, maternal self-confidence, and maternal identity.

Targeted Health Promotion Interventions

In the theme of health promotion, three studies examined the effects of yoga. Benavides and Caballero (2009 [Level III before–after study]) reported an average weight loss of 5 lbs and improvements in self-esteem for 8- to 15-year-olds at risk for Type 2 diabetes participating in a yoga program. One RCT for adolescents with irritable bowel syndrome, reported in a systematic review (Birdee et al., 2009), found reduced gastrointestinal symptoms following participation in a yoga program. Powell and colleagues (2008 [Level II nonrandomized controlled study]) reported on the effectiveness of a program of yoga, massage, and relaxation for children with behavioral difficulties and found improvements in self-confidence and increased communication compared to controls. Hernandez-Guzman, Gonzalez, and Lopez (2002 [Level I RCT]) found that a guided-imagery program with withdrawn or rejected first-graders in Mexico resulted in more socialization when imagery was combined with the rehearsal of coping strategies.

A Level I meta-analysis (Wilfley et al., 2007) provided strong evidence that lifestyle interventions, including diet, exercise, parental involvement, and self-monitoring, resulted in lower percentage of overweight in children and youth. There is moderate evidence from a Level I systematic review that participation in exergaming and educational videogames results in increased physical activity and nutritional knowledge for healthy and at-risk children (Guy, Ratzki-Leewing, & Gwadry-Sridhar, 2011).

Two Level I RCTs examined the effectiveness of training programs with children and adolescents to improve asthma self-management. In Gebert and colleagues' (1998) study, a multicomponent training program that included relaxation, social activities, and sports revealed an improvement in knowledge about asthma. McPherson, Glazebrook, Forster, James, and Smyth (2006) examined the effectiveness of an interactive computer game and found that participants in the intervention group had improved knowledge about asthma, a more internal locus of control, and fewer days off from school at 6 months compared to controls. A Level I RCT (Christian & D'Auria, 2006) evaluated the effectiveness of life skills management program for children with cystic fibrosis. Children in the intervention group had increased peer support and social competence as well as decreased loneliness at follow-up compared to the usual-care control group.

Dolgin, Somer, Zaidel, and Zaizov (1997) provided an activity-based group intervention for siblings of children with cancer in a Level III before–after study. In addition to improvements in cancer-related knowledge, participants had improved mood and communication skills.

Targeted Play, Leisure, and Recreation Interventions

The third theme for Tier 2 for the targeted interventions is play/leisure/recreation. Three studies examined the effectiveness of play for abused or neglected children (Fantuzzo et al., 1996 [Level I RCT]; Tyndall-Lynd, Landreth, & Giordano, 2001 [Level II nonrandomized controlled trial]; Udwin, 1983 [Level I RCT]). The findings indicated that play groups for this population resulted in improved play, self-esteem, and positive feelings, as well as decreased solitary play and behavior problems.

Five studies examined the impact of play and music on children with a variety of intellectual and language impairments (Duffy & Fuller, 2000 [Level I RCT]; Robertson & Weistmer, 1997 [Level I RCT]; Schery & O'Connor, 1992 [Level II nonrandomized controlled trial]; Sparling, Walker, & Singdahlsen, 1984 [Level III before–after study]; Sussman, 2009 [Level II repeated measures with participants serving as control]). Improvements were noted in social and language skills as well as attention to peers. A Level II nonrandomized controlled study examined the effects of a short-term creative program for children and early adolescents with peer difficulties (Walsh, Kosidoy, & Swanson, 1991). The results indicated an improvement in self-confidence for handling peer conflict as compared to a no-treatment control group.

The second subtheme within play/leisure/recreation is recreation, leisure, and physical education programs. Six studies examined the effects of this subtheme on children and adolescents with intellectual disabilities (Anderson & Allen, 1985a [Level I RCT], 1985b [Level I RCT]; Carter & Hughes, 2005 [Level I systematic review]; Gencoz, 1997 [Level I RCT]; Jeffree & Cheseldine, 1984 [Level III before–after study]; Santomier & Kopczuk, 1981 [Level I RCT]). The results indicated that participating in recreation, leisure, and physical education programs results in improved social interaction.

Although participants were able to learn the steps of a recreation activity, the results are inconclusive that participation in the recreation activity continued after the end of the program. A Level III before–after study examined the effect of an activity-based summer residential program for children with cleft lip and palate (Lochman, Haynes, & Dobson, 1981).

Social interaction and expectations for social interaction with peers improved at the end of the program. Lowenstein (1982 [Level I RCT]) found an increase in extraversion and a decrease in timidity following a structured recreation and activity program for children with extreme shyness compared to a control group encouraged to increase social contact. Ohl and colleagues (2008 [Level II nonrandomized controlled study]) compared participation in an activity-based after-school program for children with identified problems to children without identified problems. Although both groups improved, those with problems demonstrated a significantly greater effect size on a strengths and difficulties questionnaire than those without identified problems.

Summary: Targeted Interventions

At this level, occupational therapists, with their background in psychopathology and social participation, can play an important role in early detection, evaluation, and intervention for children and youth at risk of developing mental health challenges. Because children are generally not identified as having a mental or emotional disorder at Tier 2, evaluation efforts need to emphasize efficient but careful screening for subtle changes in behavior and/or functional skills.

A range of early intervention services focusing on promotion and prevention can be implemented, such as consultation with teachers to modify the environment or task to promote success and/or activity-based groups that focus on social skills or participation in play/leisure. Occupational therapists might collaborate with teachers, social workers, or other mental health providers to develop and cofacilitate such selective interventions.

The evidence-based review just presented provides strong support for the use of social skills programming for at-risk youth to improve social functioning and reduce problem behaviors in children and youth demonstrating antisocial behavior as well as those diagnosed with ADHD and intellectual impairment. In addition, there is strong evidence to support the use of play/recreation/leisure programming to enhance social interaction and self-esteem in at-risk groups such as children and youth with intellectual impairment, those with cleft lip/palate, and children with extreme shyness. Programs focusing on health promotion also have shown a range of positive outcomes, including improved self-esteem and social functioning and reduced symptoms in groups of children with medical challenges (e.g., diabetes, asthma, irritable bowel syndrome).

Tier 3: Intensive Mental Health Services

Intensive individualized services are provided for children and youth with identified mental, emotional, or behavioral disorders that limit participation in needed and desired areas of occupational performance. Approximately 1 in 5 children ages 9 to 17 years have a diagnosable emotional or behavioral disorder, with the most common being substance abuse disorder (10.3%), anxiety (8%), depression (5.2%), ADHD (4.5%), and conduct disorders (3.5%) (Koppelman, 2004; NRC & IOM, 2009). About half have only mild impairment and may be served by targeted services, and the other half have significant impairment. In addition, it is estimated that an average of 1 in 88 children in the United States has an autism spec-

trum disorder (ASD; Centers for Disease Control and Prevention, 2012).

Serious emotional disturbances refers to a range of diagnosable behavioral and mental disorders that severely impair daily functioning in the home, school, and community and affect approximately 5% to 9% of children and youth (U.S. Department of Health and Human Services, 1999). A greater number of children and youth in the child welfare (50%) and juvenile justice (67%–70%) systems have mental health problems (NRC & IOM, 2009). In the population of children with disabilities, it has been reported that approximately 11.5% experience psychosocial issues, with only about 42% of those actually receiving mental health services (Witt, Kasper, & Riley, 2003).

In addition to these statistics, many other children who experience social and emotional challenges that do not meet the criteria for mental health diagnosis experience impaired function and distress (Masia-Warner et al., 2006). Unfortunately, about 70% to 80% of children who need mental health services do not receive such care (Kutash et al., 2006).

At the intensive level, the person–occupation–environment transaction requires an in-depth knowledge of a range of mental health and behavioral disorders, how the disorders influence the person's functioning in a variety of occupational performance areas (e.g., education, leisure, ADLs, social participation), current medical and psychosocial interventions, and school and community services. Accessing information from reliable technical assistance centers, government reports, and current literature is essential for developing a solid knowledge base (Bazyk, 2011c).

PBS at this level takes place when targeted interventions do not meet the needs of an individual student. Intensive interventions are developed to address behaviors that are highly disruptive, dangerous, or prevent learning (Freeman et al., 2006). The process of functional behavior assessment (FBA) and behavioral intervention planning (BIP) is more time-consuming and complex at this level. An understanding of behavioral analysis and behavior management provides a foundation for this process. Tools for conducting FBAs and BIPs are available at www.pbis.org.

At the intensive level, the student's team typically includes family members, school professionals, and community members who meet regularly to develop, implement, and monitor an individualized plan of support. Occupational therapists have many opportunities to observe student behaviors in a variety of school contexts (e.g., classrooms, hallways, cafeterias, playgrounds) and thus can contribute to both the FBA and BIP processes.

Evaluation

The occupational therapist will need to use a variety of evaluation strategies to analyze the person–occupation–environment transaction and factors that are limiting occupational performance. Observations, interviews, and formal assessments are best conducted in natural school, home, and community contexts. Assessments can be broadly categorized as evaluating occupational performance and social participation. See Table 4 for examples of selected assessments.

Intervention

Although services at the intensive level are individualized to meet the specific needs of children and youth based on the mental health condition and presenting symptoms, it is critical that a systems perspective be adopted, because children and youth often benefit from supports and services that are intensive and provided by multiple systems in the community. First and foremost, interventions are occupation-based, emphasizing successful participation in occupations that the child or youth needs or wants to do in school, home, and community settings. In addition to receiving individualized services, children and youth with identified mental illness may receive and benefit from targeted Tier 2 and universal Tier 1 services.

Three key perspectives are important for guiding service provision for children and youth with mental health disorders: (1) systems of care, (2) youth empowerment, and (3) the promotion of subjective well-being. In addition, a discussion of cognitive–behavioral therapy (CBT) follows.

Systems of Care

Systems of care approaches provide a framework for youth, families, schools, and community partners to provide individualized services and supports that help children and youth with serious emotional disturbances and their families achieve their desired goals (Sebian et al., 2007). The federal entity that administers the Comprehensive Mental Health Services for Children and Their Families Program (systems of care) is the Substance Abuse and Mental Health Services Administration. Philosophies guiding systems-of-care approaches emphasize a comprehensive, integrated continuum of mental health and related services and supports that are community-based, family-driven, youth-guided, and culturally and linguistically competent.

Such approaches are necessary because youth with serious mental health disorders typically receive services from two or more public agencies, such as juvenile justice, child welfare, special education, and state and local mental health departments. Systems-of-care approaches aim to "wrap" families in a comprehensive network of community services with interagency collaboration. Coordinated services ease the burdens families may experience when services are fragmented and conflicting. Services are intended to be family-driven and youth-guided. To assist in provided comprehensive, integrated services, occupational therapy practitioners need to embrace systems-of-care approaches and work collaboratively with youth, families, and multiple service providers (Bazyk, 2011c).

Youth Empowerment

Youth involvement in systems of care begins with education and leads to opportunities for youth as decision-making partners in their own care as well as active partners in helping shape policies and procedures that govern youth in community systems of care. The youth empowerment process supports all students in becoming leaders of mental health promotion in their own lives, in their own schools, and in their communities. Youth involvement means that youth voices should be heard, valued, and utilized in all decisions that affect their lives and the lives of their peers and families (Gowen & Walker, 2009). Occupational therapy practitioners need to become aware of and support national, state, and local youth empowerment initiatives as a strategy for promoting young people's mental health.

Subjective Well-Being

Several terms have been used to describe positive thinking and feelings about one's life, including subjective well-being (Diener, 2000) and authentic happiness (Seligman, 2002). A sense of emotional well-being or happiness can be characterized by feeling and believing that one's life is satisfying and is associated with frequent experiences of positive affect, low levels of negative affect, and the ability to participate in activities that preserve these states. "Experiences that induce positive emotion cause negative emotion to dissipate rapidly" (Seligman, 2002, p. xii).

According to Seligman (2002), authentic happiness comes from identifying and developing one's *signature strengths* (i.e., strengths that are deeply characteristic of the person) and using them every day in work, love, and play. For individuals with severe and persistent mental illness and/or developmental disabilities, it is important to guard against focusing solely on the reduction of problem behaviors. Attention to participation in meaningful occupations that foster positive emotions and signature strengths will enhance a sense of emotional well-being, happiness, and quality of life.

The concept of *occupational enrichment* can be used to foster participation in occupations that promote subjective well-being and authentic happiness. Occupational enrichment involves the deliberate manipulation of the environment to support engagement in a meaningful array of occupations and is especially critical in situations involving occupational deprivation (Molineux & Whiteford, 1999).

Occupational deprivation has been described as the influence of an environment that keeps a person from developing, using, or enjoying something (Wilcock, 2006). For youth experiencing significant mental health issues or developmental disabilities, ensuring access to a range of community-based leisure occupations and supporting successful participation is recommended (e.g., arts, theater, dance, sports).

Cognitive–Behavioral Therapy

CBT is a relatively short-term, focused approach that teaches people how to modify thought patterns in order to change troublesome feelings and behavior. The emphasis is on helping the person identify cognitive distortions (inaccurate beliefs), learn effective self-help skills, and practice them in daily life (Ginsburg & Kingery, 2007).

CBT has been used with children and youth demonstrating a variety of mental health problems, including anxiety, depression, panic, posttraumatic stress disorder, and obsessive–compulsive disorder. By far, CBT is used most extensively with children who experience anxiety disorders (20%; Ginsburg & Kingery, 2007). Comorbidity among anxiety disorders and other conditions—including ADHD, oppositional defiant disorder, and ASD—is frequent; thus, CBT often is used with these populations as well (Monga, Young, & Owens, 2009).

Although CBT is primarily provided within an individual counseling framework, strategies also are typically taught to parents and other significant adults in order to promote carryover in home and school. Application of CBT at the universal, selective, and intensive levels within school contexts has also been reported (Christner, Forrest, Morley, & Weinstein, 2007). Occupational therapy practitioners need to be knowledgeable about specific CBT strategies to assist in carryover and strengthen its effectiveness. A selection of programs using CBT strategies and applied at the universal and targeted levels are presented in Table 7, along with descriptions of major CBT strategies that include psychoeducation, affective education, cognitive restructuring, relaxation training, and exposure and contingency management.

The Web site at www.schoolmentalhealth. org offers practical information on intervention approaches to address a variety of mental health conditions. The occupational risks and intervention suggestions specific to several mental health disorders are summarized in Table 8. See Box 7 for a clinical vignette of intensive interventions.

Summaries of Evidence From Systematic Reviews of Intensive Services

The focus of Tier 3 is on children and adolescents who require intensive mental health interventions. The evidence in this tier falls into two themes: (1) interventions targeted to social skill development and (2) interventions that concentrate on play, leisure, and recreation. The populations within this tier have diagnoses of mental illness, severe behavior disorders, and/or an ASD.

Intensive Social Skills Programs

Within the theme of social skills intervention, 15 studies examined children and adolescents with ASD (Aldred, Green, & Adams, 2004 [Level I RCT]; Bauminger, 2007 [Level III pretest–posttest study]; Epp, 2008 [Level III pretest–posttest design]; Kroeger, Schultz, & Newson, 2007 [Level II nonrandomized controlled study]; Laugeson, Frankel, Mogil, & Dillon, 2009 [Level I RCT]; Lee, Simpson, & Shogren, 2007 [Level I meta-analysis]; LeGoff, 2004 [Level II nonrandomized controlled trial]; LeGoff & Sherman, 2006 [Level II retrospective pre–post control, non-

randomized]; Lopata, Thomeer, Volker, Nida, & Lee, 2008 [Level I RCT]; Machalicek, O'Reilly, Beretvas, Sigafoos, & Lancioni, 2007 [Level I meta-analysis]; Mackay, Knott, & Dunlop, 2007 [Level III pretest–posttest design]; Owens, Granader, Humphrey, & Baron-Cohen, 2008 [Level I RCT]; Ozonoff & Miller, 1995 [Level II nonrandomized controlled trial]; Tse, Strulovitch, Tagalakis, Meng, & Fombonne, 2007 [Level III pretest–posttest design]; Wood et al., 2009 [Level I RCT]). The interventions studied include social skills training, self-management training, friendship skills groups, LEGO therapy, CBT, and joint attention. In general, the results indicate that social skills training has a positive impact on social behavior, social competence, and self-management, but some results were inconclusive.

Machalicek and colleagues (2007) conducted a meta-analysis of single-subject design studies of interventions used to reduce challenging behaviors in children and adolescents with an ASD and found that self-management strategies, changes in instructional content, and differential reinforcement were reported to be effective. The authors also reported that, even in studies that reported improvements in behavior, participants still demonstrated undesirable behaviors. Lee and colleagues (2007) completed a meta-analysis of single-subject design studies of self-management techniques (e.g., social skills training, self-monitoring) and found no differences with school-age children with an ASD.

Other studies reported improvements in social behaviors using specific interventions for children with an ASD. Kroeger and colleagues (2007) reported improvements in prosocial behaviors and social interaction when using video modeling or direct group instruction to deliver social skills intervention compared to free play. Laugeson and colleagues (2009) evaluated the effectiveness of a social skills training group to improve friendship skills compared to delayed treatment. The results indicated that the treatment group had better parent-reported social skills and better quality of friendship. Owens and colleagues (2008) compared a LEGO group for

Table 7. Cognitive–Behavioral Therapy (CBT) Strategies (Ginsburg & Kingery, 2007) and Examples of School Programs Using CBT

Strategy	Description
Psychoeducation Helps to demystify therapy, empower child/family, and instill hope for a positive outcome	• Educate child and family about the disorder, including typical symptoms (thoughts and bodily reactions), causes (usually multidimensional), course of treatment, and major intervention strategies. • Role of therapist as "coach." • Importance of "homework" to practice between sessions.
Affective education Helps children recognize their own and other's feelings and respond appropriately	• Teach a range of feeling words and the ability to recognize emotions through facial expressions, tone of voice, and body language. • Recognize own emotions and those of others (empathy). • Identify somatic clues related to uncomfortable emotions—anxiety (heart pounding, palms sweating, stomachache, shortness of breath); depression (fatigue, lack of energy); anger (physical tension, heart pounding). • Identify activities that influence emotions (e.g., participation in a hobby or sport can result in feelings of enjoyment and well-being).
Cognitive restructuring (reframing) Helps child learn to use self-talk to change thinking and emotions	• Recognize faulty thinking and its impact on feelings. • Identify faulty or anxious thinking and recognize why it is not realistic. • Generate coping thoughts for a situation, write them down on a card, and keep them handy. • Use "thought-stopping" strategies; replace feared thinking with less-threatening views, realistic thoughts, and positive affirmations.
Relaxation training Helps reduce feelings of anxiety and promote successful interaction and participation	• Progressive muscle relaxation teaches the difference between tense and relaxed states by tightening and relaxing muscles. The child systematically tenses and relaxes body parts to teach how to make it relax. Yoga and might meditation also might be used. • Deep breathing—Learning diaphragmatic breathing to promote relaxation. Using a balloon as a metaphor, children are instructed to put one hand on their stomach and one hand on their chest and inhale through their nose (filling stomach/chest up like a balloon), hold for 3 seconds, and exhale while imagining that they are allowing all of the anxious feelings to leave their body. • Guided imagery.
Exposure to fears and contingency management	• Explain rationale for exposure to situations—That avoiding a situation over time strengthens the avoidant response and increases anxiety; avoidance prevents the development of coping skills, the ability to succeed and gain confidence. • Exposure involves gradual introduction of the feared event, progressing from imagining situation and role playing before the actual event. • Contingency management involves rewarding brave behavior with a favored activity or small item to increase the occurrence of the behavior.

Examples of School Programs Using CBT Strategies

I Can Problem Solve Program (Shure, 2001)	• Targets violence prevention and general problem solving for children ages 4–12 years • Implemented in classroom by teacher with parent follow-through • Lessons focus on applying social problem-solving skills and creating alternative solutions to resolve conflicts using games and dialogue • Findings: Increase in prosocial behaviors, well-being, resiliency, academic concentration, as well as a decrease in stress, labels, multiple problems, and high-risk behaviors

(Continued)

Table 7. Cognitive–Behavioral Therapy (CBT) Strategies (Ginsburg & Kingery, 2007) and Examples of School Programs Using CBT *(Cont.)*

Strategy	Description
Promoting Alternative Thinking Strategies (PATHS) (Kusche & Greenberg, 1994)	• Implement at universal level within classroom. • Focuses on emotional development, self-regulation, social interaction, and social problem-solving skills. • Has been applied in both urban and rural elementary school settings. • Findings: Increased their knowledge about feelings and decreased self-reports of depression.
Anger and Aggression: Coping Power Program (Lochman & Wells, 2003)	• An evidence-based program that is designed to improve social–cognitive skills in aggressive youth. • Lessons are structured and organized and focused on specific skills that are easily taught and practiced within a school environment, such as anger management interventions, goal setting, emotional awareness, relaxation training, social skills training, problem solving, and handling peer pressure.
Anxiety/Stress: Coping Koala Program (Tomb & Hunter, 2004)	• Goal of this group program is to help children modify their frame of mind (cognitions) and experience of anxiety producing events by learning coping mechanisms. • Sessions provide the participants with skills to help handle their fears through cognitive, behavioral, and physiological coping techniques.

Note. From "Major Approaches Useful in Addressing the Mental Health Needs of Children and Youth: Minimizing Risks, Reducing Symptoms, and Building Competencies" by S. Bazyk and S. Brandenburger Shasby, in *Mental Health Promotion, Prevention, and Intervention With Children and Youth: A Guiding Framework for Occupational Therapy* (p. 67), by S. Bazyk (Ed.), 2011, Bethesda, MD: AOTA Press. Copyright © 2011 by the American Occupational Therapy Association. Adapted with permission.

children with an ASD to a social language program and a no-treatment control group. Reductions in social difficulties were reported in the LEGO group compared to the other comparison groups, and participants in the LEGO and social language groups demonstrated reductions in maladaptive behaviors.

Two studies examined the effects of a LEGO construction and social skills group on social competence in elementary-age children with autism (LeGoff, 2004; LeGoff & Sherman, 2006). LeGoff (2004) found that social initiation and duration of social interaction increased significantly for the LEGO group compared to the control group. LeGoff and Sherman (2006) reported on results of participating in a LEGO group for 3 years. The results indicated that the LEGO group improved more in social interaction than the control group. Children who initially were higher in language made greater gains during the intervention.

Wood and colleagues (2009) evaluated the effectiveness of CBT to reduce parent-reported anxiety symptoms in children with autism compared to wait-list controls. The results indicated that children in the intervention group had lower parent-reported anxiety scores at follow-up, and the authors reported a medium to large effect size, in particular for social communication skills. Epp (2008) used CBT strategies in combination with art activities and games and found a significant improvement in assertive behaviors as well as a reduction in hyperactivity and problem behaviors.

Aldred and colleagues (2004) studied a social communication intervention that included *joint attention*—the process of sharing the experience of observing an object or event by following gaze or pointing gestures—for preschoolers with autism. When compared with usual care, children in the intervention group had improvements in language and adaptive behavior. In addition, analysis of videos evaluating parent–child interaction revealed significant increases in positive synchronous communication and children communication. There was no difference in parental stress at follow-up between groups.

Table 8. Mental Illnesses, Symptoms, Performance Effects for School or Work, and Accommodations and Supports

Diagnosis	Common Symptoms	Performance Effects	Suggested Accommodations and Supports for Occupational Therapists
Thought disorders (peak age of onset is between ages 16 and 25 years)			
Schizophrenia and schizoaffective disorder	• Hallucinations—visual, auditory, olfactory, and tactile sensory distortions • Delusions—beliefs that are fixed and false • Paranoia or suspiciousness • Low registration • Reduced sense of smell • Poor insight about symptoms • Reduced ability to process information • Slowed visual scanning abilities • Mood fluctuations • Reduced facial expressions (blunting)	• Distracted by internal stimulation, making it difficult to orient to tasks and stay focused and adding to the appearance of being "odd" • Difficulty organizing thoughts and articulating well, which affects school or work performance and social relationships • Isolation and difficulties making and keeping friends because of moodiness, sensory sensitivities, suspiciousness, delayed responses, and odd behaviors • Tendency to miss key information because of poor awareness of visual cues and surroundings and slowed information processing • Difficulty reading facial expressions, which can lead to inappropriate emotional responses and poor understanding of social situations • Difficulty multitasking and understanding complex directions • May need to start at the beginning when an activity is interrupted • Suicidal thoughts and acts can be persistent, often leading to suicide completion	*Note.* Medication and other therapies may be prescribed to treat these disorders; suggestions made here are to help guide occupational therapy intervention. • Use activities to help organize thoughts and behaviors, such as deep proprioceptive tasks (e.g., calisthenics, pulling a wagon filled with soil or rocks, pushing a broom, playing tug-of-war, swinging from a rope). • Use environments with few distractions in which to perform school or work tasks, for example, quiet spaces, few interruptions, predictable changes, and not crowded. • Use clear, simple instructions that are repeated, written down, or both to ensure success; use a calm tone but not a patronizing one. • Demonstrate a new task or step first, and then allow the person to practice several times while being observed. Offer extra demonstrations and practice sessions as necessary. • Provide individualized assistance when organizing tasks, asking the person to help develop the strategies; this approach aids with recall. • Create and support opportunities for socialization with peers and coworkers, especially when social situations are not overwhelming, for example, small gatherings. Introduce client to one person who shares a common interest and assist with small talk. • Respond to signs of depression and talk of suicide. Help the person seek professional assistance when necessary.

(Continued)

Table 8. Mental Illnesses, Symptoms, Performance Effects for School or Work, and Accommodations and Supports *(Cont.)*

Diagnosis	Common Symptoms	Performance Effects	Suggested Accommodations and Supports for Occupational Therapists
Mood disorders (These disorders have multiple diagnostic variations, and not everyone experiences all the listed symptoms.) Bipolar I disorder and bipolar II disorder	Shifts in mood from sadness (depression) to elation (hypomania or mania) *Mania:* • Irritable • Decreased need for sleep • More talkative than usual • Too many ideas at once—thoughts race • Easily distracted • Poor judgment • Impulsive • Increase in goal-directed activities that may seem risky or reckless • Inflated self-esteem and ideas of special abilities • Psychomotor agitation • Delusions, hallucinations, or both (i.e., psychotic features)	*Mania:* • May react to frustration with lengthy explosive outbursts, which can lead to destruction, assault, or both • May react defiantly to authority • Can appear disorganized and scattered, leaping from one task to another with enthusiasm and sharing grand ideas but never completing anything • People associating with someone with hypomania or mania feel worn out (as though they cannot keep up) • Engage in risky behaviors, such as sexual promiscuity, overspending, reckless driving	*Mania:* • Do not engage in arguments, and call for help if the person becomes explosive, dangerous, or both. • Ignore comments about superior skills and gently encourage the person to engage in a task he or she finds meaningful. • Allow autonomy when possible. • Redirect energies to perform physical activities, either alone or with one other person (to minimize opportunities for arguments and outbursts and to help with organization of thoughts and actions). • Offer simple, structured tasks that the person finds enjoyable as a way to improve attention and focus.
Major depression	• Sadness that lingers • Irritability • Low energy • Loss of interest in activities • Difficulty initiating tasks • Sleep and appetite disturbances • Withdrawal from friends and social activities • Children and adolescents may refuse school attendance • Decreased mental functioning • Thoughts of death and suicide	• Affect appears sad, and person may not respond to or understand humor • Can appear argumentative or short tempered, which affects social relationships • Falls asleep easily, in class, at work, in social situations • May not be able to get out of bed all day • Overeats or refuses to eat, both of which are worrisome to family and friends • Difficulty starting tasks, so may fall behind at school or work • Difficulty sustaining attention with any task or activity and difficulty processing information • Difficulty making decisions • May complete suicide attempt after suicide talk or gestures	• Eliminate decision making to increase activity engagement and reduce stress. • Offer simple, structured, familiar tasks to promote self-efficacy and productivity, one at a time. • Encourage the development of daily routines that include good nutrition and some physical activity. • Advocate for shorter school and work days, with reduced tasks and expectations, even if only temporarily. • Offer to consult with employers, school personnel, and service providers to help with accommodations. • Invite participation, but do not push. • Keep conversations short and simple. • Set reasonable goals that are within the person's reach (e.g., "try doing this in the next 10 minutes"). • Be alert to signs and talk of suicide, then get help quickly.

(Continued)

Table 8. Mental Illnesses, Symptoms, Performance Effects for School or Work, and Accommodations and Supports *(Cont.)*

Diagnosis	Common Symptoms	Performance Effects	Suggested Accommodations and Supports for Occupational Therapists
Anxiety disorders (There are multiple diagnostic variations for these disorders, and not everyone experiences all the symptoms listed.) Posttraumatic stress disorder (PTSD)	• Avoiding places, people, or situations • Reexperiencing the event through images ("flashbacks"), thoughts, or perceptions • Experiencing high states of arousal, such as difficulty falling or staying asleep, irritability or outbursts of anger, difficulty concentrating, hypervigilance, exaggerated startle response • Feeling depressed or numb • Fatigue • Restlessness • Sleep disturbance because of distressing dreams of the event	• Tendency to isolate from others and withdraw from activities—may refuse school or work or drop out of extracurricular activities • Difficulty completing tasks because of fatigue, distractibility, poor concentration, restlessness, and hypervigilance • Lack of enjoyment from socializing and participating in activities • May appear fearful when asked to do something in an unfamiliar setting or with multiple people • Tends to startle easily, especially when there are loud or unexpected noises; person may have difficulty reengaging in the activity	• Explore enjoyable, calming activities, especially deep breathing, meditation, and physical exercise. • Help establish a bedtime routine that prepares for restful sleep, for example, no caffeine 5–6 hours before sleep (includes soda and chocolate), no TV 1 hour before bed, consistent bedtime. • Explore enjoyable physical activities that can be done with one other person (as a means of increasing socialization, as well). • Identify tasks the person needs to complete, then break them into easy, manageable steps with a realistic time frame (i.e., extra time allowed but within a finite period). • People may need advocacy for environmental adaptations at school or work that reduce hypervigilance.

(Continued)

Ten studies explored social skills intervention for individuals with diagnosed mental illness and/or serious behavior disorders, including schizophrenia, depression, anxiety, conduct disorders, severe behavior/emotional disorders, and alcohol and drug abuse (Amish, Gesten, Smith, Clark, & Stark, 1988 [Level II nonrandomized controlled trial]; Baker, Lang, & O'Reilly, 2009 [Level I systematic review]; Butler, Chapman, Forman, & Beck, 2006 [Level I meta-analysis]; Cook et al., 2008 [Level I meta-analysis]; Dobson, McDougall, Busheikin, & Aldous, 1995 [Level I RCT]; Gangl, 1987 [Level III before–after study]; Grizenko, Papineau, & Sayegh, 1993a [Level II cohort using repeated measures], 1993b [Level II cohort using repeated measures]; Ison, 2001 [Level I RCT]; Stermac & Josefowitz, 1985 [Level III before–after study]). The results indicates that social skill interventions improved social behaviors in these populations.

Baker and colleagues (2009) conducted a systematic review of video modeling and found that the intervention improves peer interaction and on-task behavior and reduced inappropriate behavior. Similar results were noted for the meta-analysis conducted by Cook and colleagues (2008), who reported that social skills training had a medium effect size for adolescents with serious behavior disorders, in particular for modeling, social–cognitive procedures, and operant procedures. Butler and colleagues (2006) used meta-analytic techniques to evaluate the effectiveness of CBT and found large effect sizes when CBT was used for childhood depressive and

Table 8. Mental Illnesses, Symptoms, Performance Effects for School or Work, and Accommodations and Supports *(Cont.)*

Diagnosis	Common Symptoms	Performance Effects	Suggested Accommodations and Supports for Occupational Therapists
Generalized anxiety disorder	• Excessive anxiety and worry that is difficult to control and causes disability in social, work, school, or other important areas of functioning • Feeling keyed up or on edge • Easily fatigued • Difficulty concentrating or mind going blank • Irritability • Muscle tension • Difficulty falling or staying asleep or restless, unsatisfying sleep	• Tendency to isolate from others and withdraw from activities as a way to reduce anxiety; may refuse school or work or drop out of extracurricular activities • Difficulty completing tasks because of fatigue, distractibility, poor concentration, or low frustration tolerance • May forget thoughts when talking, which increases distress • May fall asleep in school or at work • May appear restless or have difficulty engaging in tasks • May be avoided by peers because of his or her irritability • May complain of soreness in different body areas or may appear stiff during physical activities (even when walking or sitting)	• Explore enjoyable, calming activities, especially deep breathing, meditation, and physical exercise. • Identify tasks the person needs to complete, then break them into easy, manageable steps with a realistic time frame (i.e., extra time allowed, but within a finite period). Posting a daily schedule can help reduce anxiety because expectations and tasks are clear. • Discuss ways to decrease muscle tension, for example, warm baths, yoga, stretching, heating pads on muscles. • Encourage writing thoughts on paper before speaking so there is a reference and to increase confidence. • Help establish a bedtime routine that prepares for restful sleep, for example, no caffeine 5–6 hours before sleep (includes soda and chocolate), no TV 1 hour before bed, consistent bedtime. • Explore options for dealing with restlessness in socially acceptable ways at school and work, for example, asking to take a 10-minute walk break, doing gross-motor stretching. • Identify socially acceptable methods to increase arousal when sleepy in school or at work.

Sources. American Psychiatric Association (2000); Minnesota Association for Children's Mental Health (2009).
Note. From "Occupational Therapy for Youth at Risk of Psychosis and Those With Individual Mental Illness," by D. Downing, in *Mental Health Promotion, Prevention, and Intervention With Children and Youth: A Guiding Framework for Occupational Therapy* (pp. 146–147), by S. Bazyk (Ed.), 2011, Bethesda, MD: AOTA Press. Copyright © 2011 by the American Occupational Therapy Association. Reprinted with permission.

anxiety disorders. Effect sizes for childhood somatic disorders were moderate.

Intensive Play, Leisure, and Recreation Programs

The two populations studied within the theme of play/leisure/recreation were children and adolescents with ASD and studies of children with severe

behavior disorders. Five studies examined play/leisure/recreation interventions for children and adolescents with ASD (Gold, Wigram, & Elefant, 2006 [Level I systematic review]; Kim, Wigram, & Gold, 2008 [Level I RCT]; Koegel, Dyer, & Bell, 1987 [Level III before–after study]; Schleien, Mustonen, & Rynders, 1995 [Level III before–after study]; Schleien, Rynders, Mustonen, & Fox, 1990 [Level III before–after study]). Schleien and colleagues'

Box 7. Intensive Intervention—Case Study Promoting Mental Health in a Child With Autism

Occupational Profile

Hester, age 13, lives with her mother and her 9-year-old twin brothers. She was colicky as a baby, hypersensitive to changes in her food and to noises and lights, and developed language skills slowly. She often recites dialogue from movies, particularly *Beauty and the Beast*, when she feels anxious or stressed. Usually she is content to play by herself with the same few games for several hours but abandons playing when her brothers try to join her, or gets upset if the game pieces are rearranged. Her mother enjoys Hester's humor and is proud of how gentle and courageous she is.

She functions at a fifth-grade level at school, receiving all of her core instruction in a resource room. Hester participates in the general education setting for physical education, library, art, and computer instruction. Her teacher has reported instances of teasing and bullying in the hallways. When she becomes anxious or upset, she starts to moan and throws objects. This behavior has caused her peers to avoid interacting with her. She enjoys participating in ballet and tap dance class once weekly, although she does not know the name of the other girls in dance classes.

The occupational therapist meets with the Hester, her mother, and the educational team. Together, they decide that providing interventions at the Tiers 1, 2, and 3 concurrently will best educate the community about autism and support Hester's successful participation at home and in the school.

Tier 1 Interventions

The occupational therapist will do the following:
- Serve on a committee to develop a schoolwide anti-bullying initiative and to promote a positive supportive environment for all children
- Offer a 1-hour informational program about promoting social participation and positive mental health to Hester's dance instructors and be available for consultation as needed.

Tier 2 Interventions

The occupational therapist and the classroom teacher facilitate a "Circle of Friends" for Hester that includes the following:
- An initial orientation session about autism and the importance of friendship
- Monthly pizza parties with Hester and 4 girls from her class to support their efforts to encourage Hester to join them as they walk between classes and work on class projects.

The occupational therapist and speech–language pathologist will do the following:
- Organize a weekly "lunch bunch" group that includes 3 typical peers and 2 other children from Hester's resource room class to develop friendship skills
- Share with Hester's mother strategies that can be incorporated into the home to facilitate play interactions between Hester and her brothers.

Tier 3 Interventions

The occupational therapist will do the following:
- Administer 2 assessment tools (Underlying Characteristics Checklist [Aspy & Grossman, 2007] and the Individual Strengths and Skills Inventory [Aspy & Grossman, 2008]) to target specific areas to address her individualized social participation and mental health needs

(Continued)

(1990) results indicated that play activities involving higher levels of social play resulted in more appropriate levels of play behavior in school-age children with autism. A later study by Schleien and colleagues (1995) reported no change in cooperative behaviors for children with autism when paired during art activities with children without autism.

Improved social interaction by the children without autism with their peers with autism has been noted. Gold and colleagues (2006), who evaluated the effectiveness of music therapy (singing, listening to music, or playing an instrument), found a medium effect size for improvements in nonverbal communication skills and small to medium effect size for improvements in verbal communications and reductions in problem behavior. Kim and

colleagues (2008) found that improvisational music therapy that used a variety of instruments was more effective at facilitating joint attention behaviors and nonverbal social communication skills in preschoolers with autism than play.

The effectiveness of play/leisure/recreation interventions for children and adolescents with serious behavior disorders was evaluated in four studies (Grizenko et al., 1993a [Level II cohort using repeated measures], 1993b [Level II cohort using repeated measures]; Ikiugu & Ciaravino, 2006 [Level III mixed pretest–posttest with phenomenological design]; Sachs & Miller, 2001 [Level I RCT]). Ikiugu and Ciaravino (2006) used Instrumentalism in Occupational Therapy (IOT) as a conceptual guide to facilitate transition to adult-

Table 9. Examples of Occupational Therapy Intensive (Tier 3) Services

Intensive Services	School
Targeted population—Children and youth with identified • Mental health problems and/or diagnoses • Behavioral challenges • Developmental disabilities **Occupational Therapy Services** Efforts involve more direct, individualized services within a systems of care philosophy and included all of Tier 1 & II services, plus • Direct intervention (individual and group work) • Advocacy • Community integration • Consultation and collaboration • Accommodations	***Gain Knowledge*** • *Become knowledgeable about symptoms,* medical management, psychological services, and so forth, for a range of mental health disorders and how these present themselves in children and youth. • *Become knowledgeable about mental health disorders* common to children with various developmental disorders such as autism, ADHD, and intellectual disabilities. • *Identify reputable and useful Internet resources* for accessing current information about mental illness and interventions supported with evidence. ***Evaluation*** • *Evaluate school function* (classroom participation, ADLs, play/leisure, social participation, and beginning work skills) in a variety of natural contexts (classroom, lunchroom). • *Assist in the FBA process* and contribute to the development and implementation of the BIP. ***Intervention*** • *Collaborate* with the school-based mental health providers, teachers, and administrators to ensure a coordinated *system of care* for students needing intensive interventions. • *Provide ways to modify or enhance school routines* to reduce stress and the likelihood of behavioral outbursts. • *Promote the development of individual interests* by exploring extracurricular activities and providing the necessary supports to enhance successful participation. • *Offer individual or group interventions* for students with serious emotional disturbance (SED) either through special education or Section 504 to enhance participation in education, social participation, play/leisure, and ADLs. ◦ For students with ASD, consider offering the following interventions: social skills programming (Kroeger et al, 2007; Laugeson et al., 2009; Machalicek et al., 2007); LEGO® groups (LeGoff, 2004; LeGoff & Sherman, 2006; Owens et al., 2008); CBT (Epp, 2008; Wood et al., 2009); and play/leisure/recreation (Gold et al., 2006; Kim et al., 2008; Schleien et al., 1990). • For students with diagnosed mental illness, *consider offering social skills programming* (Amish et al., 1988; Baker et al., 2009; Butler et al., 2006; Cook et al., 2008; Dobson et al., 1995; Gangl, 1987; Grizenko et al., 1993a, 1993b; Ison, 2001; Stermac & Josefowitz, 1985). • *Collaborate with teachers* in modifying classroom expectations based on the student's specific behavioral or mental health needs. • *Analyze students' unique sensory needs* and develop intervention strategies to promote sensory processing and successful function in multiple school contexts (eg. classroom, cafeteria). • *Psychoeducation*: Educate teachers about the early signs of mental illness and proactive strengths-based prevention strategies. • *Provide tips* for promoting successful functioning throughout the school day, including transitioning to classes, organizing work spaces such as desk and locker, handling stress, and developing strategies for time management.

(Continued)

Table 9. Examples of Occupational Therapy Intensive (Tier 3) Services *(Cont.)*	
	Community *Gain Knowledge* • *Become knowledgeable about the health benefits* of creative arts and alternative approaches (yoga) with children and youth with mental health disorders. *Evaluation* • *Identify national and local community settings* that would welcome children and youth with identified mental health disorders (arts, theatre, music, recreation). *Intervention* • *Use coaching models* to help youth with mental health and physical challenges participate in meaningful leisure occupations.

Note. ADHD = attention deficit hyperactivity disorder; ADLs = activities of daily living; FBA = Functional Behavior Assessment; BIP = Behavioral Intervention Plan; ASD = autism spectrum disorder; CBT = cognitive–behavioral therapy.
From "Occupational Therapy Process: A Public Health Approach to Promoting Mental Health in Children and Youth" by S. Bazyk, in *Mental Health Promotion, Prevention, and Intervention With Children and Youth: A Guiding Framework for Occupational Therapy* (p. 40), by S. Bazyk (Ed.), 2011b, Bethesda, MD: AOTA Press. Copyright © 2011 by the American Occupational Therapy Association. Adapted with permission.

hood for adolescents with emotional and behavioral difficulties. IOT assists the adolescent in developing a life mission statement to organize his or her life. Strategies are then created to modify participation in areas of occupation. Although the authors reported that participation in peer-related occupations, such as talking on the phone, decreased, there was no difference in participation in leisure, education, and ADLs after involvement in the IOT program. The perceived value of family and friends improved after the IOT program. Sachs and Miller (2001) found short-term improvement in cooperation following a wilderness experience for adolescents with behavior disorders as compared to free time.

Summary: Intensive Individualized Services

Intensive individualized services are provided for children and youth with identified mental, emotional, or behavioral disorders that limit participation in needed and desired everyday activities. At this level, occupational therapy practitioners need to obtain a sound knowledge of a range of mental health disorders and how they influence the person's functioning as well as what occupation-based inter-

ventions are most effective based on evidence to support participation in context.

On the basis of the evidence available at Tier 3, there is strong support for the use of social skills programming for children with an ASD to improve social behavior, social competence, and self-management. In particular, LEGO groups for children with an ASD have been found to improve social interaction. In addition, CBT strategies have been found to improve assertive behaviors and reduce anxiety, hyperactivity, and problem behaviors in children with an ASD. There is also strong evidence that social skills interventions improve social behaviors in children and youth with mental illness and/or serious behavior disorders. The use of play activities and music has yielded positive changes in play behaviors and cooperation for children and youth with ASD; however, evidence for the use of such programs with children and youth with emotional and behavioral challenges is less conclusive.

Although not inclusive, Table 9 provides further examples of occupational therapy services at the intensive level emphasizing evaluation and intervention for children and youth with diagnosed mental health and/or behavioral challenges.

Implications for Occupational Therapy Practice, Education, and Research

The evidence in this Practice Guideline includes findings from a systematic review covering the period 1980 to 2002 as well as an updated review covering 2003 to 2009. Although the evidence from the more recent review may be more in line with a public health model for children's mental health used in this version, implications from the first edition (*Occupational Therapy Practice Guidelines for Children With Behavioral and Psychosocial Needs*) remain just as valuable. "Current best practice in occupational therapy is focused on occupation, not treatment using specific techniques or interventions in isolation. As such, occupational therapy practitioners use activities as the means to 'occupation' and for participation within a variety of contexts" (Jackson & Arbesman, 2005, p. 31).

A total of 124 articles were included in the systematic review incorporated into this Practice Guideline. The summary of the distribution of these articles is presented in Table B3. Of the articles included in the reviews, 77 were at the highest level of evidence, Level I studies. Twenty-seven articles were Level II studies, and 20 were Level III studies. When analyzing by tiers, 35 (30%) articles were in the universal tier, 57 (44%) were in the targeted tier, and 32 (26%) were in the intensive tier.

Implications for Practice

The results of the systematic review provides a wealth of evidence that supports an individual client impairment-focused model of practice; targeted services for at-risk groups; and population, strengths-based approaches. The evidence also provides support for an occupation- and activity-based approach that can be used at all three levels in a wide range of environments (e.g., school, home, community) and contexts. Table 10 lists general recommendations based on the evidence previously mentioned in this Practice Guideline.

The results at the universal level indicate that there is strong evidence for occupational therapy practitioners to provide occupation- and activity-based interventions in many areas. The evidence is strong, for example, that activity-based emotional-learning programs improve social skills and that schoolwide programs prevent bullying and victimization. Activity-based problem-solving skills programs also have been shown to improve coping behavior in children. Occupational therapy practitioners working in after-school programs should consider incorporating a social skills component, because the evidence is strong that these activities-based interventions improve social behaviors and reduce problem behaviors. In the area of health promotion, school-based stress management programs have been shown to reduce stress and improve coping skills in children in grades three through eight.

At the universal level, occupational therapy practitioners also can play a role in improving participation in play/leisure/recreation. The evidence is

(Continued on p. 70)

Table 10. Recommendations for Occupational Therapy Interventions for Mental Health Promotion, Prevention, and Intervention for Children and Youth

Recommended*	No Recommendation	Not Recommended
Tier I		
Social Skills Interventions		
• Whole-school and emotional learning programs to improve social and emotional skills (A) • After-school programs incorporating a goal of social skills to improve social behaviors and reduce problem behaviors (A) • School-based bullying prevention programs to prevent bullying and victimization (A) • Problem-solving skills to improve coping behavior (A) • Problem-solving skills to improve peer interaction in preschool-age children (B) • Parent education to improve child compliance (B) • Parent education as part of a multicomponent school program to prevent aggressive behaviors in at-risk kindergartners (B)		
Health Promotion		
• School-based stress management programs for Grades 3–8 to reduce stress and improve coping skills (A) • Mental health literacy programs for adolescents to improve knowledge and attitudes about mental illness (B) • Back education program for elementary school children to improve back posture when lifting objects and carrying backpacks (B) • Yoga to improve physical fitness and cardiorespiratory health (B or A) • Yoga to reduce negative behaviors in response to stress (C)	• School-based programs to improve self-efficacy (I)	
Play/Recreation/Leisure		
• Participation in performing arts programs to improve social interaction and social skills (A) • Use of recreation facilitators in after-school programs to increase participation in physical activity (B) • Participation in performing arts programs to reduce emotional problems (B) • Team-building activities during physical education to improve self-concept (B) • Teaching cooperation skills in elementary school children to increase cooperation and reduce competitive behaviors (B) • Skill-based activity groups to reduce involvement with the legal system (C) • Skill-based activity groups to improve behavioral outcomes (I)	• Bike repair program for adolescents to improve self-esteem and ability to work with others (I)	

(Continued)

Table 10. Recommendations for Occupational Therapy Interventions for Mental Health Promotion, Prevention, and Intervention for Children and Youth *(cont.)*

Recommended*	No Recommendation	Not Recommended
Tier II		

Social Skills

- Social skills training for disliked or rejected children and adolescents to improve social interaction, peer acceptance, and social standing (A)
- Social skills programming for at-risk, aggressive, or antisocial children and adolescents to improve attention to tasks, peer interaction, and prosocial behaviors and to reduce aggressive, delinquent, and antisocial behaviors (A)
- Social skills programming for children and adolescents with learning disabilities and ADHD to improve communication and social and functional skills and reduce problem behaviors (A)
- Social and life skills programs for children with intellectual impairments and developmental delays to improve life skills, conversation turn-taking, initiation of social interaction, self-management, and compliance, and to decrease problem behaviors (A)
- Parenting programs for teenage mothers and their children to improve mother–infant interaction and parental attitudes and knowledge, maternal mealtime communication, self-confidence, and identity (A)

Health Promotion

- Yoga for adolescents with irritable bowel syndrome to reduce gastrointestinal symptoms (A)
- A program of yoga, massage, and relaxation for children with behavioral difficulties to improve self-confidence and increase communication (B)
- A guided-imagery program combined with coping strategies for withdrawn or rejected first graders to increase socialization (B)
- A multicomponent training program for children and adolescents with asthma to improve knowledge of asthma and internal locus of control and to decrease days off from school (B)
- Yoga for youth with Type 2 diabetes to increase weight loss and self-esteem (C)
- An activity-based group intervention for siblings of children with cancer to improve cancer-related knowledge, mood, and communication skills (C)

(Continued)

Table 10. Recommendations for Occupational Therapy Interventions for Mental Health Promotion, Prevention, and Intervention for Children and Youth *(cont.)*

Recommended*	No Recommendation	Not Recommended
Play/Recreation/Leisure		
• Play groups for abused or neglected children to improve play skills, self-esteem, and positive feelings and to reduce solitary play and behavior problems (A) • Play and music for children with intellectual and language impairments to improve social skills and attention to peers (A) • Recreation, leisure, and physical education programs for children and adolescents with intellectual disabilities to improve social interaction (A) • Structured recreation and activity program for children with extreme shyness to increase extraversion and decrease timidity (B) • Creative activities for children and early adolescents with peer difficulty to improve self-confidence in managing peer conflict (C) • Activity-based summer program for children with cleft lip and palate to improve social interaction (C) • Activity-based after-school program for children with identified behavior problems to improve self-concept (C)		
Tier III		
Social Skills		
• Social skills training for children and adolescents with ASD to improve social behavior, social competence, and self-management (A) • LEGO® social skills group for children with ASD to reduce social difficulties and improve social interaction (A) • Social skills interventions for individuals with diagnosed mental illness and/or serious behavior disorders to improve social behaviors (A) • Friendship skills group for children with ASD to improve social skills (B) • Cognitive–behavioral therapy for children with ASD to reduce parent-reported anxiety (B)		

(Continued)

Table 10. Recommendations for Occupational Therapy Interventions for Mental Health Promotion, Prevention, and Intervention for Children and Youth *(cont.)*

	Recommended*	No Recommendation	Not Recommended
	• Social communication intervention that includes joint attention for preschoolers with autism to improve language and adaptive behavior (B) • Cognitive–behavioral therapy and activities and games for children with ASD to improve assertive behavior and reduce hyperactivity and problem behaviors (C) • Video modeling or direct group instruction in social skills for children and adolescents with ASD to improve prosocial behaviors and social interactions (C) • Self-management strategies, change in instructional content, and differential reinforcement for children with ASD to reduce challenging behaviors (I)		
Play/Recreation/ Leisure			
	• Music-related activities (singing, listening to music, playing an instrument) for children with autism to improve nonverbal and verbal communication skills and reduce problem behaviors (A) • Wilderness experiences for adolescents with behavior disorders to improve cooperative behaviors (B) • Play activities for school-age children with autism to increase play and cooperative behaviors (I) • Use of a program to identify life mission (Instrumentalism in Occupational Therapy) for adolescents with emotional and behavioral difficulties to improve participation in occupations (I)		

The terminology used for the recommendations was language used in the article(s) from which the evidence was derived.

Note. Criteria for level of evidence (A, B, C, I, D) are based on standard language of Agency for Healthcare Research and Quality (2009). Suggested recommendations (recommended, no recommendation, not recommended) are based on the available evidence and content experts' clinical expertise regarding the value of using the intervention in practice.

ADHD = attention deficit hyperactivity disorder; ASD = autism spectrum disorder.

A—There is strong evidence that occupational therapy practitioners should routinely provide the intervention to eligible clients. Good evidence was found that the intervention improves important outcomes and concludes that benefits substantially outweigh harm.

B—There is moderate evidence that occupational therapy practitioners should routinely provide the intervention to eligible clients. At least fair evidence was found that the intervention improves important outcomes and concludes that benefits outweigh harm.

C—There is weak evidence that the intervention can improve outcomes, and the balance of the benefits and harms may result either in a recommendation that occupational therapy practitioners routinely provide the intervention to eligible clients or in no recommendation, because the balance of the benefits and harm is too close to justify a general recommendation.

I—Insufficient evidence to determine whether or not occupational therapy practitioners should be routinely providing the intervention. Evidence that the intervention is effective is lacking, of poor quality, or conflicting, and the balance of benefits and harm cannot be determined.

D—Recommend that occupational therapy practitioners do not provide the intervention to eligible clients. At least fair evidence was found that the intervention is ineffective or that harm outweighs benefits.

(Continued from p. 65)
strong, for example, that participation in performing arts programs improves social interaction and social skills. A recent report by the Catterall, Dumais, and Hampden-Thomson (2012) indicated that children and adolescents from low-socioeconomic-status backgrounds who participate in arts programming either at school or in extracurricular programs achieve better success in school.

At the targeted level, there is strong evidence that social and life skills programs are effective for a wide range of at-risk children, such as those who are aggressive or rejected and those who are teenage mothers. There is also strong evidence that play groups for abused or neglected children improve play skills and reduce behavior problems. In addition, there is strong evidence that children with intellectual impairments, developmental delays, and learning disabilities would benefit from social skills programming and play, leisure, and recreational activities. Occupational therapy practitioners are the ideal professionals to provide this type of programming, because they have a wealth of knowledge of both the challenges these groups of children and adolescents face as well as of activity-based programming.

In the area of health promotion, the evidence that adolescents with irritable bowel syndrome benefit from yoga to reduce gastrointestinal symptoms is moderate. Although not typically seen in a school-based setting, occupational therapy practitioners should consider community-based yoga programming for this population.

The evidence for the effectiveness of social skills programs is also strong for children who require services at the intensive level. These occupation- and activity-based programs are effective in helping children with an ASD improve social behavior and self-management. In addition, social skills programs are effective in improving social behaviors for children and adolescents with diagnosed mental illness and/or serious behavior disorders.

Implications for Education

Occupational therapy academic programs have a long history of incorporating mental health practice into curricula. Occupational therapy practitioners are well prepared not only to recognize mental health problems but also to understand how to assess and provide intervention to children and youth needing intensive services. The information provided in this Practice Guideline, however, takes a broader approach in emphasizing mental health promotion and prevention interventions for children and youth without diagnosed mental illness.

It is important for academic programs and fieldwork education to prepare students to apply a public health model of children's mental health at the universal, targeted, and intensive levels in both school- and community-based practice. The evidence-based practice guidelines ensure that the expansion into a public health model can be explored while maintaining an occupation- and activity-based approach.

Implications for Research

Although much of the evidence to date, as reported in this Practice Guideline, was published by researchers outside the field of occupational therapy, it is critical for occupational therapy practitioners to use this existing evidence to support practice as described in each tier. For example, when developing new programs focusing on social skills, play/leisure/recreation, or health promotion, summaries of evidence provided can be used to document the benefits of such programs.

In addition, occupational therapy practitioners need to be committed to generating evidence to support services provided at the universal, targeted, and intensive levels. At the universal level, they may want to collaborate with teachers and administrators in assessing school climate or whole-class SEL following the implementation of whole-school programming. Collecting pre- and posttesting of social skills when implementing small-group interventions to targeted at-risk students is another example of obtaining evidence to evaluate intervention outcomes. Finally, clear documentation of student outcomes when providing individualized services provides evidence regarding the effects of intervention for individual students. Occupational therapy practitioners also can agree to collaborate in any large-scale RCTs conducted at their setting.

Appendix A. Preparation and Qualifications of Occupational Therapists and Occupational Therapy Assistants

Who Are Occupational Therapists?

To practice as an occupational therapist, the individual trained in the United States
- Has graduated from an occupational therapy program accredited by the Accreditation Council for Occupational Therapy Education (ACOTE®) or predecessor organizations;
- Has successfully completed a period of supervised fieldwork experience required by the recognized educational institution where the applicant met the academic requirements of an educational program for occupational therapists that is accredited by ACOTE or predecessor organizations;
- Has passed a nationally recognized entry-level examination for occupational therapists; and
- Fulfills state requirements for licensure, certification, or registration.

Educational Programs for the Occupational Therapist

These include the following:
- Biological, physical, social, and behavioral sciences

- Basic tenets of occupational therapy
- Occupational therapy theoretical perspectives
- Screening evaluation
- Formulation and implementation of an intervention plan
- Context of service delivery
- Management of occupational therapy services (master's level)
- Leadership and management (doctoral level)
- Professional ethics, values, and responsibilities.

The fieldwork component of the program is designed to develop competent, entry-level, generalist occupational therapists by providing experience with a variety of clients across the lifespan and in a variety of settings. Fieldwork is integral to the program's curriculum design and includes an in-depth experience in delivering occupational therapy services to clients, focusing on the application of purposeful and meaningful occupation and/or research, administration, and management of occupational therapy services. The fieldwork experience is designed to promote clinical reasoning and reflective practice, to transmit the values and beliefs that enable ethical practice, and to develop professionalism and competence in career responsibilities. Doctoral-level students also must complete a doctoral experiential component designed to develop advanced skills beyond a generalist level.

Who Are Occupational Therapy Assistants?

To practice as an occupational therapy assistant, the individual trained in the United States

- Has graduated from an occupational therapy assistant program accredited by ACOTE or predecessor organizations;
- Has successfully completed a period of supervised fieldwork experience required by the recognized educational institution where the applicants met the academic requirements of an educational program for occupational therapy assistants that is accredited by ACOTE or predecessor organizations;
- Has passed a nationally recognized entry-level examination for occupational therapy assistants; and
- Fulfills state requirements for licensure, certification, or registration.

Educational Programs for the Occupational Therapy Assistant

These include the following:
- Biological, physical, social, and behavioral sciences
- Basic tenets of occupational therapy

- Screening and assessment
- Intervention and implementation
- Context of service delivery
- Assistance in management of occupational therapy services
- Professional ethics, values, and responsibilities.

The fieldwork component of the program is designed to develop competent, entry-level, generalist occupational therapy assistants by providing experience with a variety of clients across the lifespan and in a variety of settings. Fieldwork is integral to the program's curriculum design and includes an in-depth experience in delivering occupational therapy services to clients, focusing on the application of purposeful and meaningful occupation. The fieldwork experience is designed to promote clinical reasoning appropriate to the occupational therapy assistant role, to transmit the values and beliefs that enable ethical practice, and to develop professionalism and competence in career responsibilities.

Regulation of Occupational Therapy Practice

All occupational therapists and occupational therapy assistants must practice under federal and state law. Currently, 50 states, the District of Columbia, Puerto Rico, and Guam have enacted laws regulating the practice of occupational therapy.

Note. The majority of this information is taken from the *2011 Accreditation Council for Occupational Therapy Education (ACOTE) Standards* (ACOTE, 2012).

Appendix B.
Evidence-Based Practice

One of the greatest challenges facing health care systems, service providers, public education, and policymakers is ensuring that scarce resources are used efficiently. The growing interest in outcomes research and evidence-based health care over the past 30 years, and the more recent interest in evidence-based education, can in part be explained by these system-level challenges in the United States and internationally. In response to the demands of the cost-oriented health care system in which occupational therapy practice is often embedded, occupational therapists and occupational therapy assistants are routinely asked to justify the value of the services they provide on the basis of scientific evidence. The scientific literature provides an important source of legitimacy and authority for demonstrating the value of health care and education services. Thus, occupational therapy practitioners, other health care practitioners, and educators increasingly are called on to use the literature to demonstrate the value of the interventions and instruction they provide to clients and students.

According to Law and Baum (1998), *evidence-based occupational therapy practice* "uses research evidence together with clinical knowledge and reasoning to make decisions about interventions that are effective for a specific client" (p. 131). An evidence-based perspective is founded on the assumption that scientific evidence of the effectiveness of occupational therapy intervention can be judged to be more or less strong and valid according to a hierarchy of research designs or an assessment of the quality of the research. AOTA uses standards of

evidence modeled on those developed in evidence-based medicine. This model standardizes and ranks the value of scientific evidence for biomedical practice using the grading system in Table B.1 (Sackett, Rosenberg, Muir Gray, Haynes, & Richardson, 1996). In this system, the highest levels of evidence include systematic reviews of the literature, meta-analyses, and randomized controlled trials (RCTs). In RCTs, the outcomes of an intervention are compared with the outcomes of a control group, and participation in either group is allocated randomly. The systematic reviews presented here include Level I RCTs; Level II studies, in which assignment to a treatment or a control group is not randomized (cohort study); and Level III studies, which do not have a control group.

The evidence-based literature review undertaken for this Practice Guideline examined studies that evaluated the effects of activity-based intervention on peer and social interaction, compliance with adult directives and social rules and norms, or productive or task-focused behavior in individuals from ages 3 to 21 years at the universal, targeted, and intensive tiers. These topics were chosen by a consensus group of clinical experts, because it was felt that these areas were the most representative of the psychosocial components that predict participation in school and in the home and community. In other words, on the basis of expert opinion, children who were able to interact in peer and social environments and/or comply with adult directives and engage in task behavior were more likely to successfully participate in school and in the home and community environments.

Table B.1. Levels of Evidence for Occupational Therapy Outcomes Research

Level of Evidence	Definitions
Level I	Systematic reviews, meta-analyses, randomized controlled trials
Level II	Two groups, nonrandomized studies (e.g., cohort, case control)
Level III	One group, nonrandomized (e.g., before–after, pretest–posttest)
Level IV	Descriptive studies that include analysis of outcomes (e.g., single-subject design, case series)
Level V	Case reports and expert opinion that include narrative literature reviews and consensus statements

Note. Adapted from "Evidence-Based Medicine: What It Is and What It Isn't" by D. L. Sackett, W. M. Rosenberg, J. A. Muir Gray, R. B. Haynes, and W. S. Richardson, 1996, *British Medical Journal, 312*, pp. 71–72. Copyright © 1996 by the British Medical Association. Adapted with permission.

The following focused question was included in the review:

What is the effectiveness of activity-based interventions for mental health promotion, prevention and intervention with children and youth? The interventions include those focused on peer and social interaction; compliance with adult directives and social rules and norms; and participation in productive and task-focused behavior.

To conduct the evidence-based literature review, reviewers evaluated research studies published in the peer-reviewed scientific literature according to their quality (scientific rigor and lack of bias) and levels of evidence. The evidence-based reviews incorporated into the AOTA Practice Guidelines consist of a review and ranking of the literature relevant to occupational therapy interventions published since 1980 used to treat a variety of clinical conditions. An initial review covered articles published between 1980 and 2002 (Jackson & Arbesman, 2005). An updated review included articles published between 2003 and 2009. In addition, more recent articles covering the period 2010 to 2012 were included on the basis of recommendations from content experts in the field. Specific inclusion criteria were as follows:

- The article was published either in a peer-reviewed journal or in a peer-reviewed evidence-based review since 1980 in the English language.

- The age range of study participants was 3 to 21 years.
- The intervention described in each study was embedded in activities and within the domain of occupational therapy, although it did not have to be a common occupational therapy intervention or administered by an occupational therapist or an occupational therapy assistant.
- The outcomes measured in the study included social or peer interactions or compliance with adult directives or social rules and norms.
- Level I, II, and III evidence.

Exclusion criteria were the following:

- Presentations and conference proceedings
- Non–peer-reviewed literature
- Dissertations and theses
- Study did not include an activity-based component
- Study was outside the scope of occupational therapy practice
- Level IV and V evidence.

Reviewers and AOTA staff first identified search terms, and these were reviewed by the advisory group. The search terms were developed not only to capture pertinent articles but also to make sure that the terms relevant to the specific thesaurus of each database were included. Table B.2 lists the search terms related to populations and interventions included in each systematic review. For the updated review, additional search terms were added to reflect changes in terminology that had taken

Table B.2. Search Terms

Search Terms for Original Search (1980–2002)

Activities, activities of daily living, activity groups, adaptation, adaptive behavior, aggression, alcohol, anger management, antisocial behavior, approach, behavior, behavior(al) disorders, bullying, communication skills training, conflict resolution, cooperative behavior, coping strategies, craft, decision-making skills, disruptive behavior disorders, drug, emotional support, emotionally disturbed, exercise, experiential learning, family, field trip, friendship, games, group activities, health, human activities, impulsive behavior, instrumental activities of daily living, interaction, interpersonal, intervention, job training, leisure, mental disorders, mental health, outcome management, peer group, peer interaction, personal care, physical, physical education, play, pregnancy prevention, prevocational, problem solving, program effectiveness, prosocial development, psychiatric, psychological, psychosocial, recreation, reinforcement, religion activities, resistance skills, reward, role, self-care, self-concept, sexual activity, sibling support, social behavior disorders, social competence, social skills, specialized interventions, sports, stress, substance abuse prevention, support, tasks, teaching, team, therapy, token economy, treatment, treatment effectiveness

Additional Search Terms For Follow-up Search (2003–2009)

Activities, character strengths, community integration, coping skills, delayed gratification, flow, graded activity, group process, health, hobbies, homeless children, impulse control, impulsivity, interest development, interpersonal, juvenile delinquency, learning, managing emotions, mental health promotion, organized activities, out-of-school activities, participation, positive behavioral, positive mental health, positive psychology, prevention of psychosis, promotion/wellness, public health approach, relationships, resiliency, school mental health, school violence, self-calming, self-advocacy, self-determination, social emotional, social participation, structured leisure, supports, systems of care, transition, work/vocational

place since the earlier review. Search terms for the updated reviews were developed by the consultant to the AOTA Evidence-Based Practice Project and AOTA staff in consultation with the author of the questions and were reviewed by the advisory group. A medical research librarian with experience in completing systematic review searches conducted all updated searches.

The following sources were searched:

- Bibliographic databases (MEDLINE, ERIC, Embase, PsycINFO; OTseeker was included in the updated review)
- Consolidated information sources (e.g., evidence-based medicine reviews, including the Cochrane Database of Systematic Reviews, the Cochrane Controlled Trials Register, and the Database of Abstracts of Reviews of Effectiveness).

The AOTA consultant completed the initial review of the database results. The updated review was completed by an academic partnership of Susan Nochajski and master's students in occupational therapy at the University at Buffalo, State University of New York. The team of reviewers also scanned the bibliographies of selected key articles. After the literature search, reviewers then evaluated the quality of the studies and ranked them using the evidence-based standards described in Table B.1.

The teams working on the focused question reviewed the articles according to their quality and levels of evidence. Each article included in the review then was abstracted using an evidence table that provides a summary of the methods and findings of the article and an appraisal of the strengths and weaknesses of the study based on design and methodology. AOTA staff and the evidence-based practice project consultant reviewed the evidence tables to ensure quality control. All studies identified by the review, including those not specifically described in this section, are summarized in Appendix C. (Readers are encouraged to read the full articles for more details.)

A total of 124 articles were included in the earlier and updated reviews. Although the reviews included published literature from occupational therapy and related fields, all studies provided evidence within the scope of occupational therapy practice. Seventy-seven of the articles (62%) were classified as Level I evidence, 27 of the articles

Table B.3. Number of Articles in Each Tier at Each Level of Evidence

Review	Evidence Level					Total in Each Review
	I	II	III	IV	V	
Tier 1	26	7	2	0	0	35
Tier 2	36	13	8	0	0	57
Tier 3	15	7	10	0	0	32
Total	77	27	20	0	0	124

(22%) were classified as Level II studies, and 20 (16%) were classified as Level III studies. Table B.3 shows the distribution of the articles by level and tier.

The articles included in the systematic review have several overarching limitations, including the following: small sample size; wide variation in interventions, diagnoses, and clinical conditions; wide variation in outcomes measured; and the use of self-report outcome measures. Depending on the level of evidence, there may have been a lack of randomization, lack of control group, and limited statistical reporting. A wide range of diagnoses and clinical conditions may have been included in meta-analyses and systematic reviews incorporated in these reviews.

Appendix C.
Evidence Tables

Table C.1. Universal Programs

Author/Year	Study Objectives	Level/Design/ Participants	Intervention and Outcome Measures	Results	Study Limitations
Berger et al. (2009)	To examine the effect of yoga on the well-being of children in the inner city.	Level II—Nonrandomized control group. $N = 72$ inner-city 4th- and 5th-graders in an after-school program $n = 39$ in a yoga class $n = 32$ in a non-yoga class	Intervention: Yoga group for 4th- and 5th-grade students in an after-school program Control: Non-yoga program for 4th- and 5th-grade students in an after-school program Outcome Measures: • Harter's Global Self-Worth and Physical Appearance subscales • Perceptions of Physical Health • Yoga teachings (Negative Behaviors, Positive Behaviors, and Focusing/ Relaxation subscales).	Children in the yoga group had better postintervention Negative Behaviors scores and balance than those in the non-yoga group. There were no differences for global self-worth and perceptions of physical well-being.	Yoga intervention was of short length. Lack of randomization
http://dx.doi.org/10.1016/S088-2006(96)90010-1					
Bhavnagri & Samuels (1996)	To investigate whether children's literature supported by activities with peer-related concepts could facilitate social cognition by peer relationships in preschoolers.	Level 1—Randomized controlled trial. 22 participants in experimental group, 22 participants in control group. Mean age—4 years, 3 months (range 3–5 years).	Experimental condition: 15 stories with peer-related concepts read and discussed, followed by activities to reinforce concept. Control condition: 15 stories read that had other themes (e.g., fall and Halloween activities) related to concept. Outcome Measure: Social Knowledge Interview—Children asked what characters could do in given situation.	Children in group using children's literature supported by activities with peer-related concepts had significantly higher scores on social cognition of peer relationships (relationship enhancing, assertiveness, effectiveness, relevancy) than those in control group.	Separate contributions of reading children's literature and engagement in follow-up activities could not be identified. Unknown whether improvement of social cognition resulted in shifts in behavior. No long-term follow-up
Birdee et al. (2009)	To evaluate the effectiveness of yoga among the pediatric population.	Level 1—Systematic review. Database search included CINAHL, Cochrane, EMBASE, Medline, PsycINFO, and manual search of retrieved articles.	34 controlled studies from 1979–2009 were retrieved on the effects of yoga on physical fitness, motor skills/strength, mental health, and irritable bowel syndrome. Outcome Measures: • Balance, fine motor, hand grip, mood, anger, fatigue, anxiety • Functional disability and gastrointestinal symptoms.	There is limited evidence that yoga is effective in improving physical fitness and mental health. There is limited evidence that yoga reduces gastrointestinal symptoms in adolescents with irritable bowel syndrome.	The authors reported that the included studies had methodological limitations, which limits the strength of the evidence.
http://dx.doi.org/10.1016/j.acap.2009.04.002					

Study	Purpose	Design	Results	Limitations
Bosworth et al. (1998)	To examine effects of SMART Talk, a computer-based violence prevention intervention for young adolescents.	Level III—Before–after. 98 7th graders (45% boys, 55% girls) from small city middle school with diverse social-economic population.	SMART Talk computer program engaged adolescents in games, simulation, cartoons, animation, and interactive interviews. Outcome Measures: • Teen Conflict Survey in pre- and posttest • Computer use about computer program.	SMART Talk was popular among young adolescents, and its use increased self-knowledge, conflict management skills, and practice of prosocial behaviors.	Lack of control group makes it difficult to determine if results were due to normal development or computer program.
Cardon et al. (2002) http://dx.doi.org/10.1097/00007632-200202010-00020	To evaluate efficiency of 6-session back education program in elementary school.	Level II—Nonrandomized controlled trial. Intervention: 198 participants in Practical test, 38 in Candid camera, 347 in Questionnaire. Control group: 165 participants in Practical test, 31 in Candid camera, 349 in Questionnaire. Ages 9–11 years.	Back education program with 10 guidelines used to attain good body mechanics and correct posture while participants performed various tasks in class. Outcome Measures: • Practical test measured movement in different tasks • Candid camera used observation during a lesson in classroom and movement • Questionnaire investigated back and neck pain.	Back education was effective in reducing back and neck pain for elementary school children when tested after 1 week, 3 months, and 1 year.	Lack of random assignment.
Conduct Problems Prevention Research Group (2002)	To examine longitudinal effects of Fast Track, a conduct-problem prevention trial for children grades 1 to 3.	Level I—Randomized controlled trial. Controlled with whole school assignment. 445 students assigned to Fast Track, 446 to control. Mean age 6.5 years.	Schools randomized to either universal intervention that included social and emotional development curriculum or universal curriculum plus parent groups; social skills training that included films, stories, and role-plays; home visiting; and academic tutoring. Outcome Measures: Measures of child conduct problems, social cognition, academic progress, social competence, and parenting behavior.	Though no significant effects were noted for academic progress and social competence, evaluation at 3 years' post-trial indicated that children in intervention were significantly less likely to exhibit evidence of serious conduct problems than control children. Control children were more likely to receive a special education diagnosis than intervention children.	Given extensive nature of treatment protocol, one must be careful when analyzing impact of activity-based intervention.

(Continued)

Table C.1. Universal Programs

Author/Year	Study Objectives	Level/Design/ Participants	Intervention and Outcome Measures	Results	Study Limitations
Daykin et al. (2008)	To evaluate the effects of performing arts on adolescent health and behavior.	Level I—Systematic review. 17 electronic databases were searched.	Interventions in the review included music, performance, drama, and dance in community settings and noncurricular mainstream education. Outcome Measures: · Social skills · Well-being · Knowledge of health-related topics · Self-expression · Drug use.	14 articles were included in the review, and all focused only on drama. Although outcomes were positive in all areas, the strongest outcomes were for peer interaction and social skills.	Wide variation in outcomes and study design
http://dx.doi.org/10.1177/1359105307086699					
DeMar (1997)	To examine effectiveness of school-based preventive intervention on personal and social competencies for students.	Level II—Before–after with control group. 57 students from chemically dependent or at-risk families (36 students in intervention group, 21 in control group). Ages 8–12 years.	Social group work intervention consisted of social skills training (including videotapes and games) and cognitive problem-solving in substance abuse prevention. Outcome Measures: · Personal and social competencies by Self-Concept Attitudinal Inventory · Norwicki–Strickland Locus of Control Scale · Teacher–Child Rating Scale.	Social–cognitive group intervention focused on substance abuse prevention was more effective than control group in increasing students' internal locus of control, frustration tolerance, and assertive social skills and in decreasing acting-out behavior.	Lack of random assignment.
Durlak et al. (2010)	To evaluate the effectiveness of after-school programs (ASPs) to promote personal and social skills in children and adolescents.	Level I—Meta-analysis. Searched Medline, PsycINFO, ERIC, and Dissertation Abstracts International as well as manual searches of 3 journals and reference lists of articles.	75 reports including 69 different programs were reviewed. ASPs were defined as programs that had 1 or more activities that (a) occurred during at least part of the school year, (b) happened outside of normal school hours, and (c) were supervised by adults. In addition, the program included personal or social skill development. Outcome Measures: · Feelings and attitudes—Child self-perceptions and bonding to school · Behavioral adjustment—Positive social behaviors, problem behaviors, and drug use · School performance—Achievement test scores, grades, and school attendance.	Participants in an ASP demonstrated significant increases in self-perceptions and bonding to school, positive social behavior, school grades, and levels of academic achievement, as well as significant reductions in problem behaviors compared to controls.	Many included studies lacked data on racial and ethnic composition or socioeconomic status of participants. Limited long-term follow-up Multiple categories of outcome measures
http://dx.doi.org/10.1007/s10464-010-9300-6					

Author/Year	Purpose	Design/Search	Sample/Outcome Measures	Results	Limitations
Durlak et al. (2011)	To evaluate the effectiveness of school-based universal social and emotional learning (SEL) programs for students in kindergarten through high school.	Level I—Meta-analysis. Searched Medline, PsycINFO, and Dissertation Abstracts International as well as manual searches of 11 journals and review of reference lists of articles.	213 studies of SEL programs for children and adolescents without any identifiable adjustment or learning problem. Outcome Measures: • Social and emotional skills • Attitudes toward self and others • Positive social behaviors • Conduct problems • Emotional distress • Academic performance.	SEL participants demonstrated significantly improved social and emotional skills, attitudes, behavior, and academic performance	Only one third of studies assessed skills as an outcome. Limited studies gathered data on academic achievement.
http://dx.doi.org/10.1111/j.1467-8624.2010.1564.x					
Ebbeck & Gibbons (1998)	To investigate effectiveness of Team Building Through Physical Challenges (TBPC) program on self-conceptions of physical education students in grades 6 and 7.	Level I—Randomized controlled trial. 120 students in grades 6 and 7 (58 boys, 62 girls). Mean age 11.4 years (range: 10–12 years).	8-month TBPC program included 22 physical challenges. Students in treatment group completed regular daily physical education curriculum and 1 TBPC activity every second week. Students in control group completed regular physical education curriculum without any TBPC activities. Outcome Measures: 6 items in self-concept by Self-Perception Profile for Children.	TBPC had a positive impact on self-concept of physical education students.	Other factors such as academic curriculum, extracurricular activity, and family background were not considered in analysis.
Galantino et al. (2008)	To evaluate the effect of yoga on the quality of life and physical outcome measures in the pediatric population.	Level I—Systematic review. Databases reviewed included Medline, EMBASE, CINAHL, PsycINFO, PEDro, and Cochrane.	Included 24 case control, pilot, cohort, and randomized controlled trials that examined yoga as an exercise intervention for children Outcome Measures: • Quality of life • Cardiorespiratory fitness • Physical functioning.	Yoga is effective in improving cardiorespiratory function, grip strength, flexibility, and body composition. The results of studies of neuromuscular function are inconclusive.	Small number of trials included in the review that had significant results.
http://dx.doi.org/10.1097/PEP.0b013e31815f1208					

(Continued)

Table C.1. Universal Programs

Author/Year	Study Objectives	Level/Design/ Participants	Intervention and Outcome Measures	Results	Study Limitations
Geldhof et al. (2007)	To evaluate the effects of a back education program for elementary school children at a 2-year follow-up.	Level I—Randomized controlled trial, randomized at school level. $N = 398$ 4th- and 5th-grade children at 2-year follow-up $n = 98$ intervention $n = 101$ control	Intervention: Back education program, basic principle of posture, and movement breaks. Control: No intervention. Outcome Measures: • Year 1 & 2—Knowledge of back education sessions and how frequently postural behaviors are used • Year 2—Supplemental questions on postural behavior.	At the 2-year follow-up, more children in the intervention group reported that they had integrated favorable biomechanical back posture principles when lifting and sitting compared to controls.	Use of self-report High dropout rate Potential introduction of back education separate from intervention
http://dx.doi.org/10.1007/s00586-006-0227-4					
Jones & Offord (1989)	To compare effectiveness of 2 recreational programs—traditional Boys & Girls Club and PALS (Participate and Learn Skills)—on skills of low-income children in leisure activities and on reducing antisocial behavior.	Level II—Cohort–nonrandomized controlled trial. 417 in PALS program, 488 in Boys & Girls Club. Ages 5–15 years. All living in publicly funded apartments in Canada.	PALS program offered activities in 25 recreational areas (e.g., hockey, dance, guitar). Boys & Girls Club offered open recreational activities but no outreach services. Outcome Measures: • PALS program records pre- and postintervention measured skills in performance areas and integration of activities in community • Connors Teacher Rating Scales • Connor Parent Rating Scales • Piers–Harris Children's Self-Concept Scales measured impact on behavior in school and community.	Children in PALS program increased their skill levels and had some integration into community activities, particularly in community hockey. Although no differences existed on behavioral measures, significantly fewer police charges were made against juveniles, and there were fewer security violations in PALS group.	Lack of random assignment
http://dx.doi.org/10.1111/j.1469-7610.1989.tb00786.x					

Author (Year)	Study Objectives	Level/Design/Participants	Intervention and Outcome Measures	Results	Study Limitations
Kinnevy et al. (1999) http://dx.doi.org/10.1300/J009v22no1_03	To evaluate short-term effects of different levels of participation in highly motivating activities-based group interventions for low-income youth.	Level II—Nonrandomized controlled trial. 21 participants with low incomes; 18 boys, 3 girls. Ages 9–12 years (mean age 10 years).	Participants assigned to 1 of 3 groups: graduates of an Earn-A-Bike program, waiting to start program, or current participants in program. Earn-A-Bike program included 6 highly structured sessions where participants learned bicycle safety skills and basic bicycle repair, completed 8 hours of community service, and passed an examination before graduating and receiving a bicycle. Outcome Measures: • Self-esteem and ability to work with others by self report • Problematic behavior by days of missing school and self-assessment.	Although there were no significant differences in outcomes among groups, intervention seems to improve practical and social skills, and participants benefited from positive adult role models.	Measures were limited to self-reports and measures of school attendance and disciplinary measures at school.
Kraag et al. (2006) http://dx.doi.org/10.1016/j.jsp.2006.07.001	To evaluate the effect of school programs targeting stress management or coping skills in school children.	Level 1—Meta-analysis. Participants were in grades 3–8. Databases searched included ERIC, PsycINFO, Cochrane, Medline, and Google.	Randomized and quasi-experimental controlled studies were included in the analysis. Studies received an intervention of relaxation training, social problem solving, social adjustment, and emotional self-control, or a combination of these interventions. Outcome Measures: • Adjustment and coping • Self-efficacy • Problem solving • Heart rate variability • Knowledge of stress.	19 studies were included in the meta-analysis. Although there were positive effects for reducing stress symptoms and enhancing coping skills, there was no effect for self-efficacy.	Heterogeneity of effects The authors reported that studies with positive effects are published more frequently, indicating publication bias.

(Continued)

Table C.1. Universal Programs

Author/Year	Study Objectives	Level/Design/ Participants	Intervention and Outcome Measures	Results	Study Limitations
Kutnick & Brees (1982)	*Study I* To test effects of exercises related to cooperation. *Study II* To look at effects of cooperative tasks in relation to spontaneous play.	*Study I* Level I—Randomized controlled trial. 15 participants in experimental group, 13 in control group. Ages 4.9–5.3 years. 18 boys, 10 girls. *Study II* Level II—Nonrandomized controlled trial. 6 participants from nursery class in experimental group, 6 in control group. Ages 4–5 years. 6 boys, 6 girls.	*Intervention—Study I* During free-play periods, experimental groups jointly participated in exercises, including equal and opposite forces, see-saw, rocking, and a blind walk; control group maintained free play. *Study II* Experimental children cooperatively played together with puzzles, drawing, towers, etc., whereas control group maintained normal free play activities. Outcome Measures: • Cognitive—Observation of cooperation and competition during a testing session (table-top 3 × 3 grids construction). • Moral—2 pictures chosen to evaluate children's awareness of others and reactions in an interpersonal dilemma.	*Study I* Children in experimental group showed less competitive and more cooperative behavior on cognitive task and more child–child responses in moral interview. *Study II* There were no significant differences on cognitive test or moral interviews.	Small sample size in Study II. Reliability and validity of outcome measures not reported in either study.

http://dx.doi.org/10.1111/j.2044-8279.1982.tb02522.x

Author/Year	Study Objectives	Level/Design/ Participants	Intervention and Outcome Measures	Results	Study Limitations
Lefebvre-Pinard & Reid (1980)	To assess efficacy of social conflict and modeling as methods for teaching communication skills.	Level I—Randomized controlled trial. 40 typical children; 20 boys, 20 girls. Mean age 6 years 8 months (range 5 years 2 months–8 years 11 months).	All participants randomly assigned to 1 of 5 groups: group 1 (social conflict), group 2 (modeling), group 3 (conflict–modeling) group 4 (no feedback), and group 5 (control). Plastic-covered cards were used in tasks. Outcome Measures: Communication skills by role-taking task and referential communication task in pretest, posttest, and 2-month follow-up. Measure materials included 94 plastic-covered cards with pictures of children, fruits, animals, or familiar objects.	Social conflict and modeling showed positive effects on communication skills for typical children. Social conflict and modeling together did not appear to be more effective in enhancing children's performances than either method alone.	Validity of outcome measure not reported.

http://dx.doi.org/10.2307/1129605

Citation	Purpose	Study Design/Sample	Intervention/Outcome Measures	Results	Limitations
McMahon et al. (2000) http://dx.doi.org/10.1016/S092-1849(00)80004-9	To compare effectiveness of violence prevention programs with young, at-risk children in two settings.	Level III—Before–after. 56 preschool children (ages 3–5 years) 53 kindergarten children (ages 4–7 years).	Violence prevention program, "Second Step" (for pre-K to 8th grade), used to decrease aggressive behavior and increase prosocial behavior. Each lesson includes introductory activity (usually puppets and role-playing). Outcome Measures: · Child interviews · Teacher ratings · Behavioral observations pre- and posttest.	Preschoolers and kindergarteners demonstrated significant gains in knowledge based on interview scores and significant decrease in problem behaviors based on behavior observations. Teacher rating did not change over time.	No control group; difficult to determine if results were due to normal development or teacher effects. A relatively small and transient sample.
McNeil et al. (2009) http://dx.doi.org/10.14278/ajhp.071010107	To evaluate the effectiveness of outreach support to increase school-age children's participation in recreational activities.	Level I—Cluster randomized controlled trial. 16 of 17 schools were randomized to the following conditions: $n = 6$ control $n = 5$ home-based $n = 5$ school-based $n = 360$ in Grades 3–5 in a section of Alberta, Canada, with high unemployment.	Interventions: Recreation facilitators or connectors worked with children and families in both school- and home-based settings to help children engage in more recreational activities. Control condition: Current standard of self-directed activity. Information given to intervention groups was kept in a binder in control classrooms and parents were reminded twice about the binder. Outcome Measures: · Children's Assessment of Participation and Enjoyment (CAPE) · Physical and psychosocial health, coordination, self-esteem.	A greater proportion of children in the intervention group compared to the control group increased participation in physical activity at follow-up. There were no differences between groups on a skill-based activity subscale. Children who increased their activity were more likely to have higher levels of contact with the connectors.	29% of eligible families articipated in the study. Connectors were not blinded to group assignment. First use of the CAPE as a longitudinal measure

(Continued)

Table C.1. Universal Programs

Author/Year	Study Objectives	Level/Design/ Participants	Intervention and Outcome Measures	Results	Study Limitations
Mulcahy & Schachter (1982)	To compare treatment effects of cognitive self-modeling, conversational group counseling, and no-treatment group on interpersonal skills for adolescent students.	Level I—Randomized controlled trial. 97 students; 36 boys, 61 girls. Mean age 16.5 years. All participants randomly assigned to Cognitive Self-Modeling (*n* = 39), Conventional Group Counseling (*n* = 40), or No-Treatment Control (*n* = 41).	Guided symbolic rehearsal tasks in Cognitive Self-Modeling training used to restructure each participant's existing network of cognitions or associations related to interpersonal skills. Participants in Conventional Group Counseling encouraged to communicate with members and use role-playing for teaching purposes. Outcome Measures: • Interpersonal skills measured by Personality Inventory, Self-Disclosure Questionnaire, Trait Ratings, Behavior Ratings • Background Information • Questionnaire in pretest, posttest, 10-week follow-up, and 1-year follow-up.	Both Cognitive Self-Modeling and Conventional Group Counseling were more influential in enhancing interpersonal functioning than was no treatment.	Reliability and validity of outcome measures not described in study.
Pinto-Foltz et al. (2011)	To evaluate the effectiveness of a program to improve mental health literacy and reduce stigma.	Level I—Cluster-randomized controlled trial. *N* = 156 girls ages 13–17 *n* = 95 intervention groups *n* = 61 control groups	Intervention: "In Our Own Voice," a program that provides knowledge about mental illness and facilitates intergroup contact with persons with mental illness Control group: No intervention Outcome Measures: • Revised Attribution Questionnaire—mental illness stigma • "In Our Own Voice" Knowledge Measure—Mental health literacy.	Mental health literacy was improved at 4- and 8-week follow-up for those in intervention group. There was no difference between groups for mental illness stigma.	Dose and duration of intervention may not have large enough to demonstrate a change.
Serna et al. (2000)	To determine whether children receiving self-determination program would perform better on mental health–related outcome measures than those receiving standard mental health services.	Level I—Randomized controlled trial. 84 participants—53 in experimental group, 31 in control group. Mean age 4.5 years. Children identified as being behavioral risk through teacher nomination and score on aggression measure	Classroom-wide universal intervention on direction following, sharing, and problem solving was embedded in a story and song format for participants. Outcome Measures: • Social Skills Rating System–Teacher Form, Early Screening Project • Vineland Screener, IOWA Conners • Children's Global Assessment Scale for measuring mental health functioning.	Children in experimental group who were at risk for development of emotional or behavioral disorders before intervention either significantly improved or maintained preintervention functioning of mental health as noted by adaptive behavior, social interaction, and attention measures.	Small sample size Lack of a systematic method to assess fidelity of treatment Preliminary nature of universal intervention

Author (Year)	Purpose	Design/Level/Sample	Intervention/Outcome Measures	Results	Limitations
Stevahn et al. (2000)	To evaluate knowledge and behavioral changes due to conflict resolution training program for kindergarten children.	Level 1—Randomized controlled trial. 41 experimental group (19 in morning class, 22 in afternoon class), 39 control group. Kindergarten students.	Daily conflict resolution training consisting of what is and is not conflict and 6-step negotiation process. Children engaged in activities designed to help them learn negotiation steps. Control group used same instructional material related to friendship concepts that also was included in experimental program. Outcome Measures: Interviews on conflict scenarios, negotiation conflict scenarios, medical conflict, friendship, and negotiation frequency tally.	Children receiving conflict resolution training were more likely than control group children to not only have learned integrative negotiation procedure, but also appeared to internalize it.	None.
http://dx.doi.org/10.1111/1467-8624.00184					
Tankersley et al. (1996)	To evaluate effects of school-based early intervention program to prevent antisocial behaviors that could lead to onset of conduct disorder.	Level 1—Randomized controlled trial. 34 participants in experimental group, 11 in control group. Mean age 56 months. Children nominated by teachers as being at risk for developing conduct disorders.	Prevention program included affection activities (large group activities to encourage social interaction), group activities in social skills instruction, and structured play experience to encourage generalization. Outcome Measures: • Definition for social interaction • Multiple Option Observation System for Experimental Studies • Direct observation of social behavior.	Students in experimental group demonstrated significantly lower levels of disruptive behaviors, interacted with others, and complied with teacher directions more than those in control group.	Intervention program was in place for only 4 months. Given number of components to intervention, it is difficult to separate the impact of any 1 intervention. Small sample size for control group
http://dx.doi.org/10.1177/106342669600400304					
Ttofi & Farrington (2009)	To evaluate the effectiveness of anti-bullying programs in schools.	Level 1—Meta-analysis. Published and unpublished reports of anti-bullying programs since 1983—randomized and nonrandomized controlled studies with samples of 200 or greater.	Of 600 reports located, only 59 (describing 30 programs) were eligible for inclusion. Programs included whole-school anti-bullying programs, classroom management, information for teachers and parents, and teacher training. Outcome Measures: Instances of bullying and victimization.	School-based anti-bullying programs reduced bullying and victimization by 20%–23% compared to control schools. The most effective programs included parent education, work with peers, classroom rules, and classroom management.	Analysis was not done for subgroups of participants.
http://dx.doi.org/10.1108/17596599200900003					

(Continued)

Table C.1. Universal Programs

Author/Year	Study Objectives	Level/Design/ Participants	Intervention and Outcome Measures	Results	Study Limitations
Tuttle et al. (2006)	To evaluate the effectiveness of adding a component called Positive Adolescent Life Skills (PALS) training to preexisting intervention for reducing risk-taking behaviors in teenagers.	Level 1—Randomized controlled trial with pre/posttest. *N* = 16 (10 males, 6 females) 12- to 16-year-olds without developmental delay attending an urban secondary school.	Intervention in the PALS group included structured cognitive–behavioral life skills training with focuses on basic communication, positive social participation, and problem-solving skills. Control: Teen club, a group intervention that includes health education, community outreach, and assistance. Outcome Measures: • Problem Oriented Screening Instrument for Teenagers (POSIT) • Group interviews.	There was no statistically significant difference between the intervention and control group.	Small sample size limited statistical power. The POSIT is a self-report assessment, which limits reliability of results. Cost–benefit analysis of the program does not support this intervention for the length that it was conducted.
	http://dx.doi.org/10.1016/j.pedhc.2005.10.011				
Vaughn & Ridley (1983)	To evaluate effectiveness of interpersonal problem-solving program on social behavior for preschool children.	Level 1—Randomized controlled trial. 22 in experimental group, 22 in control group. Ages 4–5 years, matched for age, gender.	Experimental group: Problem-solving training session included components of interpersonal problem model and used cognitive strategies, modeling, and role-playing. Control group: Reading or telling stories through use of puppets. Outcome Measures: Behavioral observation of quantity and quality of behavior by target child toward peers and adults.	Children in problem-solving program demonstrated significant increase in positive verbal and nonverbal peer interaction compared to those in control group.	Lack of follow-up assessment
Vreeman & Carroll (2007)	To evaluate the effectiveness of school-based interventions to reduce bullying.	Level 1—Systematic review. The following databases were searched: MEDLINE, PsycINFO, Embase, ERIC, Cochrane, Physical Education Index, and Sociology: A SAGE Full-Text Collection.	Of 2,090 articles located, 26 met inclusion criteria. The interventions included curriculum, multidisciplinary, whole-school, social skills groups, and mentoring. Outcome Measures: • Direct: Bullying, victimization, aggressive behavior, and school responses to violence • Indirect: School achievement, perceived school safety, self-esteem, and knowledge or attitudes toward bullying.	Four of 10 curriculum studies demonstrated decreased bullying, but in 3 of those 4 the decrease was not across all populations. Of 10 whole-school approach studies, 7 studies showed positive effects with greater effects for older than younger children. Mentoring programs demonstrated reduced bullying.	Limited number of search terms for review—used only *bullying and bully*.
	http://dx.doi.org/10.1001/archpedi.161.1.78				

Citation	Purpose	Design	Outcome Measures	Results	Limitations
Wahler & Meginnis (1997) http://dx.doi.org/1207/s15394424jccp2604_12	To teach mothers to provide praise and mirroring contingent on their children's positive behavior.	Level 1—Randomized controlled trial. 36 children without disabilities and their mothers; 12 dyads in each group. Mean age 7.45 years for children, 35.84 years for mothers.	Mothers in mirroring and praise group participated in 15-minute training sessions; control mothers spent 15 minutes with a trainer who simply asked about typical social interactions. Mothers asked to structure play time around game of pick-up sticks. Outcome Measures: • Psychological adjustment of mothers and children by Bell Object Relations–Reality Testing Inventory and Child Behavior Checklist • Mother–child interactions by Standardized Observation Codes–Revised • Assessment measure developed for study.	Training mothers in appropriate use of mirroring or praise could facilitate higher percentage of child compliance and higher rating of dyadic satisfaction for experimental groups.	Lack of follow-up assessment
Walker et al. (1998) http://dx.doi.org/10.1177/106342669800600201	To investigate effect of First Step to Success as an early intervention for preventing school antisocial behaviors of at-risk kindergarteners.	Level 1—Randomized controlled trial. 24 kindergarteners in experimental group (1993–1994), 22 in waitlist control group (1994–1995). 26% were girls.	All children exposed to First Step to Success early intervention program—screening, school intervention, and parent/caregiver training for supporting and improving child's school performance. Outcome Measures: • Social interaction and participation and education measured by teacher ratings of adaptive behavior maladaptive behavior • Academic engagement time observations from early screening project Aggression subscale and withdrawal subscale from teacher rating form.	First Step to Success was successful in moving target students to within normative range on aggression scales. Statistically significant improvements also were noted for target participants on teacher-rated behavioral levels at postintervention and follow-up.	Use of a wait-list control group unable to account for influence of time, setting, secular trends, and other extraneous factors.

(Continued)

Table C.1. Universal Programs

Author/Year	Study Objectives	Level/Design/ Participants	Intervention and Outcome Measures	Results	Study Limitations
Walsh-Bowers & Basso (1999)	To examine improvement of peer relations in 7th grade students through creative drama.	Level II—Cohort-nonrandomized controlled group. Intervention 1 (rural setting)—20 in intervention class (aggressive with peers and teachers) and control class (typical class). Intervention 2 (urban setting)—29 in intervention class (students with social skills deficits), 49 in control class (typical children). 7th grade.	In both interventions, students participated in 15-week drama program that included warm-up exercises, modernized fairy-tale enactments, and realistic skits. Outcome Measures: • Peer Interaction Scale (PIS) • Peer Evaluation Inventory (PEI) • Parent Ratings of Social Skills (PRSS) • Group Satisfaction Scale (GSS).	In rural school program, intervention class showed equivalent progress of peer-relation on self-report, whereas parents reported greater progress. In urban setting, students improved on teacher measure of peer problems but fell behind on teacher measure of peer strengths. Improvement in peer relations skills appear to have been partially achieved through drama program.	Intervention and comparison roups not equivalent Intervention period of limited length Some students perceived drama groups as punitive.

http://dx.doi.org/10.1080/02615470120106997

Author/Year	Study Objectives	Level/Design/ Participants	Intervention and Outcome Measures	Results	Study Limitations
Waters et al. (2011)	To update the previous Cochrane review of childhood obesity prevention research and determine the effectiveness of evaluated interventions intended to prevent obesity in children.	Level I—Meta-analysis. The searches were rerun in CENTRAL, MEDLINE, Embase, PsycINFO, and CINAHL in March 2010.	Outcome Measures: • Prevalence of overweight, obesity • Weight and height • Percentage fat content • Body mass index (BMI).	There is strong evidence that childhood obesity prevention programs affect BMI, particularly for children ages 6 to 12 years. Promising strategies for occupational therapy practitioners include developing a school curriculum that includes healthy eating, physical activity, and body image; increased physical activity and movement skills during school; environments and cultural practices to support healthy eating and increased physical activity; and providing support to teachers and parents to increase healthy eating and physical activity.	Some studies included in the meta-analysis had small sample sizes. Heterogeneity of studies included in the review

http://dx.doi.org/10.1002/14651858.CD001871.pub3

Author (Year)	Purpose	Design/Method	Intervention and Outcome Measures	Results	Limitations/Comments
Wells et al. (2003)	To evaluate the effectiveness of universal approaches for mental health promotion and disease prevention programs in schools.	Level I—Systematic review. Databases searched included MEDLINE, PsycLIT, ERIC, CINAHL, and Embase. Search completed in 1999.	Interventions were provided to the general school population and were provided completely or in part at the school. The aim of the interventions was to promote some aspect of mental health or prevent mental illness or behavior problems. Outcome Measures: • Self-concept • Behavior problems • Social problem-solving strategies • Assertiveness • Depression • Anxiety.	Seventeen studies summarizing 16 interventions were included. There was a positive effect of universal approaches for programs that adopted a whole-school approach, were implemented continuously for more than a year, and were focused on the promotion of mental health as opposed to the prevention of mental illness.	A great deal of variety of included interventions and outcome measures

http://dx.doi.org/10.1108/09654280310485546

Author (Year)	Purpose	Design/Method	Intervention and Outcome Measures	Results	Limitations/Comments
Wright et al. (2006)	To evaluate the effectiveness of a structured arts programs in low-income communities. 9/15	Level II—Nonrandomized controlled trial. N = 183 9- to 15-year-olds in 5 low-income communities across Canada. Control group matched to intervention from the National Longitudinal Survey of Children and Youth (NLSCY).	Interventions: After sessions exploring a variety of art media, the remaining sessions focused on team preparation of either a theatrical performance or a video production. Outcome Measures: Taken from NLSCY— • Behavioral and classroom observation • Self-report of conduct problems • Hyperactivity, conduct problem, and emotional problem measures.	Observer ratings showed significant gains in artistic and social skills. Comparisons with matched controls using estimated linear propensity scores revealed a significant reduction in emotional problems for the intervention group.	Intervention and comparison groups not equivalent. Intervention period of limited length. Some students perceived drama groups as punitive.

http://dx.doi.org/10.1177/0272431605285717

Table C.2. Targeted Interventions

Author/Year	Study Objectives	Level/Design/Participants	Intervention and Outcome Measures	Results	Study Limitations
Anderson & Allen (1985a) http://dx.doi.org/10.1016/0005-7967(85)90176-7	To determine effects of leisure education program on people with mental retardation.	Level I—Randomized controlled trial. 40 residents of state residential facility for people with mental retardation. Mean age 35 years (range 13–64 years).	Experimental group participated in Joswiak's leisure education program that included a variety of activities (e.g., sewing, table games, sports), guided discovery, role-play techniques—2 sessions per week over 9 weeks. Control group: Followed daily routine with assurance of nonparticipation in treatment. Outcome Measures: • Observation of social interactions • Activity involvement with staff and peers.	Leisure education program had a positive effect on frequency of activity involvement but no effect on duration of activity involvement and frequency and duration of social interaction. Duration of involvement was affected by level of retardation.	Short intervention period to reveal effects of treatment
Anderson & Allen (1985b)	To estimate effect of recreation therapy program on activity involvement and social interaction of people with mental retardation.	Level I—Randomized controlled trial. 64 participants (55 men, 9 women) with mental retardation. Mean age 33 years (range 16–65 years).	All participants randomly assigned to a treatment group with 10-week recreation therapy program and control group with regular daily schedule. Outcome Measures: Frequency and duration of social interaction and activity involvement of participants.	Recreation therapy program did not result in a significant increase of activity involvement and social interaction of individuals with mental retardation.	Treatment period may be insufficient to change participants' behavior patterns.
Antia & Kreimeyer (1996)	To examine effect of social skills or integrated-activities intervention on social interaction and acceptance of deaf or hard-of-hearing children and their peers.	Level II—Nonrandomized controlled trial. 91 normally hearing children, 45 deaf or hard-of-hearing children, ages 4–6 years: 1. Social-skills intervention: 25 deaf or hard-of-hearing children, 27 normally hearing children 2. Integrated-activities intervention: 20 deaf or hard-of-hearing children, 21 normally hearing children 3. 43 untrained normally hearing children.	All participants assigned to small groups (4–8 children in each group; half were deaf or hard-of-hearing) that received social-skills intervention or integrated-activities intervention. Outcome Measures: • Social interaction by videotape during free-play sessions • Social acceptance by a rating scale of peer photographs.	1. Social-skills intervention increased interaction between deaf or hard-of-hearing children and their deaf or hard-of-hearing peers. Treatment effects were maintained 4 weeks after intervention ceased. Neither intervention increased interaction between deaf or hard-of-hearing and normally hearing peers. 2. Neither intervention increased normally hearing children's social acceptance of deaf or hard-of-hearing peers, but increased recognition.	Lack of random assignment Systematic data on peer interaction during intervention not obtained.

94   Mental Health Promotion, Prevention, and Intervention for Children and Youth

Study	Purpose	Design	Intervention/Outcome Measures	Results	Limitations
Benavides & Caballero (2009) http://dx.doi.org/10.1016/j.ctcp.2008.12.004	To evaluate the effectiveness of a yoga program to reduce weight in youth at risk for developing type 2 diabetes.	Level III—Before–after study. $N = 20$ children, primarily Hispanic, from ages 8–15 enrolled. 14 completed the program.	Intervention: Ashtanga yoga (power yoga) program for youth at risk of developing type 2 diabetes. Outcome Measures: • Weight • Self-concept • Anxiety • Depression.	The average weight loss was 2 kg. Four of five children with low self-esteem improved, although two had decreases in self-esteem. Symptoms of anxiety were reduced at the completion of the program.	Small sample size Lack of control group Few biochemical measures assessed
Bierman & Furman (1984) http://dx.doi.org/10.2307/1129841	To examine effects of social-skills training and peer involvement on peer acceptance of disliked preadolescents.	Level I—Randomized controlled trial. 28 boys, 28 girls (5th and 6th graders) low in peer acceptance and conversational skills.	All participants randomly assigned to conversational skills training, peer involvement with group experience, conversational skills training and peer involvement with group training, and no treatment. Outcome Measures: • Observation of conversational skills • Children's knowledge by Conversational Skill Concept Scale • Social Self-Efficacy Scale.	Conversational skills training while making a film promoted skills acquisition and increased skillful social interaction. Peer involvement in group activity of making a film promoted peer acceptance and children's self-perceptions of their social efficacy.	Participants randomized to 1 of 4 groups, yielding a small sample size. Not reported if evaluators were blind to treatment condition at follow-up.
Bierman et al. (1987) http://dx.doi.org/10.1037/0022-006X.55.2.194	To investigate effects of social-skills training with instructions and/or prohibitions for improving social behavior and peer acceptance of rejected boys.	Level I—Randomized controlled trial. 32 boys who were rejected by peers based on sociometric nomination and negative social behavior.	Each target child engaged in cooperative activities (e.g., art, games) and randomized to 1 of 4 conditions: instructions to promote positive social behavior, prohibitions to reduce negative behavior, combination of instructions and prohibitions, no treatment. Outcome measures: • Aggression ratings (Pupil Evaluation Inventory—Peer and Teacher Rating) • Sociometric status—boys rated how much they liked playing with given classmate.	Prohibitions for negative behaviors resulted in immediate and stable declines in negative behavior and led to temporary increases in positive responses received from peers. Interactions and reinforcement of specific social skills promoted sustained, positive peer interactions 6 weeks after treatment. Combination of instructions and prohibitions led to improved sociometric ratings from non-target treatment partners.	Small sample size of treatment/no treatment groups

(Continued)

Table C.2. Targeted Interventions

Author/Year	Study Objectives	Level/Design/Participants	Intervention and Outcome Measures	Results	Study Limitations
Birdee et al. (2009) http://dx.doi.org/10.1016/j.acap.2009.04.002	To evaluate the effectiveness of yoga among a pediatric population.	Level I—Systematic review. Databases search included CINAHL, Cochrane, Embase, MEDLINE, PsycINFO, and manual search of retrieved articles.	34 controlled studies from 1979–2009 were retrieved on the effects of yoga on physical fitness, motor skills/strength, mental health, and irritable bowel syndrome. Outcome Measures: • Balance • Fine motor and hand grip • Mood, anger, fatigue, anxiety • Functional disability and gastrointestinal symptoms.	There is limited evidence that yoga is effective in improving physical fitness and mental health or that yoga reduces gastrointestinal symptoms in adolescents with irritable bowel syndrome.	The authors reported that the included studies had methodological limitations, which limits the strength of the evidence.
Carter & Hughes (2005) http://dx.doi.org/10.2511/rpsd.30.4.179	To determine the efficacy of interventions aimed at increasing social interaction between adolescents in secondary school with intellectual disabilities and their peers.	Level I—Systematic review. N = 109 participants with intellectual disabilities; 47% female, 40% male, gender not provided for remaining 13% Ages: 11–22 years (M = 15)	Intervention: 12 of 27 articles considered skill-based (activity-based). Most interventions utilized some variation of a structure that used modeling, practicing, prompting, praise, and corrective feedback in role-playing activities, computer games, and recreational/leisure activity. Outcome Measures: Although no specific outcome measures were listed, the following were listed as outcomes: social interaction, social contacts, social initiation, turn-taking.	Skill-based interventions resulted in improvements in discrete social skills: initiations, responses, conversational turn-taking, and social interactions at varying degrees for a wide range of severity levels (mild to profound). Effects of skill-based interventions were maintained in all studies at a follow-up period of 2–8 weeks. Improvements noted in eye gaze, reciprocity, expansions, and conversational topics. Communication book instruction and social interaction skill instruction were most effective for participants with severe impairment.	Limited information regarding participants' level of communication skills, problematic behaviors, and speech mode for many studies, which limits generalizability. Multiple contextual variables among studies: Extent to which these variables influenced outcomes of programs is unclear. Small sample sizes Long-term effects not reported

Author (Year)	Purpose	Design / Sample	Intervention / Outcome Measures	Results	Limitations
Charlebois et al. (1999)	To examine effectiveness of social skills and self-regulation skills training on boys who display inattentive, overactive, and aggressive behavior.	Level III—Before–after. 30 boys with inattention and aggressive behavior (mean age 6 years). 15 from families of low socioeconomic status, 15 from middle-class families.	An after-school program, "The Friendship Club," which included free play, self-regulation activities (problem solving through craft activities) and social-skills training. Sessions were videotaped and analyzed by trained researchers. Outcome measures: Behaviors analyzed included disobedience, sustained attention, bullying, destroying objects, and cooperating.	Participants were more able to have sustained attention during self-regulation tasks postintervention than preintervention. There was no difference in other behaviors.	One-third of participants did not complete program. Outcome measures not standardized.
Christian & D'Auria (2006)	To test the effectiveness of teaching children with cystic fibrosis (CF) life skills for management of CF using an intervention to improve psychosocial adjustment, functional health, and physiologic health.	Level 1—Randomized controlled trial. $N = 116$ children with CF $n = 58$ intervention $n = 58$ control Ages 8–12 years	Intervention: Building CF Life skills Intervention (BLS) Group sessions focused on problem solving and social skills and individual sessions tailored to each child's needs Control: Usual care Outcome Measures: • Perceived Illness Experience Scale • Self-Perception Profile for Children • Social Support Scale for Children, Children's Loneliness Scale • Functional Disability Inventory for Children • Pulmonary function and physical growth.	Those in the BLS group had decreased perceived impact of illness and decreased loneliness that was maintained throughout follow-up. Peer support from peers, scholastic competence, social competence, and behavior conduct improved over time for those in the BLS group. Global self-worth was significantly greater for those in BLS group, but both improved over time.	Most participants had mild CF severity. 9-month intervals may not be sufficient to reveal changes in development and illness.
			http://dx.doi.org/10.1097/00006199-200609000-00002		
Conduct Problems Prevention Research Group (2007)	To evaluate the effectiveness of the Fast Track Program in preventing antisocial behavior and psychiatric disorders among kindergarteners at high and moderate levels of risk.	Level I—Randomized controlled trial. $N = 891$ kindergarteners at 4 sites at high and moderate risk randomly assigned by matched sets of schools $n = 445$ intervention $n = 446$ control	Interventions: Fast Track—10 year included parent behavior management training, child social cognitive skills training, reading tutoring, home visiting, mentoring, and a universal classroom curriculum. Control: Treatment as usual. Outcomes Measures: • NIMH Diagnostic Interview Schedule for Children at grades 3, 6, and 9 • Self-report of delinquency after grades 6 and 9.	Those at high initial risk and participating in the Fast Track intervention had fewer diagnoses for conduct disorder, attention deficit hyperactivity disorder, and any externalizing disorders and lowered anti-social behavior scores. Effects were detected at grade 3 and continued through grade 9.	Because this was a multicomponent study, it is unknown if specific components are more effective than others. Unknown if effects will last through adulthood.
			http://dx.doi.org/10.1097/chi.0b013e31813e5d39		

(Continued)

Table C.2. Targeted Interventions

Author/Year	Study Objectives	Level/Design/Participants	Intervention and Outcome Measures	Results	Study Limitations
Coren & Barlow (2001) http://dx.doi.org/10.1002/14651858.CD002964	To examine the effectiveness of individual- and/or group-based parenting programs in improving psychosocial and developmental outcomes in teenage mothers and their children.	Level I—Systematic review. Cochrane review that searched MEDLINE, Embase, CINAHL, PsychLIT, Sociofile, Social Science Citation Index, ASSIA, the Cochrane Library (including SPECTR), CENTRAL, National Research Register, and ERIC for RCTs.	Four studies were included in the review of individual and group-based parenting programs. Outcome Measures: Mother–infant interaction, language development, parental attitudes, parental knowledge, maternal mealtime communication, maternal self-confidence, and maternal identity.	Individual- and group-based parenting programs resulted in positive outcomes for teenage mothers and their children.	Small number of studies included in review Limited number of outcomes measured
Csapo (1986)	To investigate effects of social-skills training on neglected and rejected children.	Level I—Randomized controlled trial with multiple baseline design. 20 neglected, 20 rejected children (28 boys, 12 girls). Ages 7.9–8.9 years.	Participants assigned to experimental group (play games with social-skills training) and attention control group (play games without social skills instruction). Outcome Measures: • Sociometric rating by peers, teacher ratings by Social Withdrawal Subscale of Walker Problem Behavior Behavior Checklist • Negative and Positive Social Behavior Subscales of Social Behavior Rating Scale • Direct observation of social interaction with peers.	Social-skills training had a positive impact for neglected and rejected children on their sociometric status, social behavior, and social interaction with peers.	Validity and reliability of assessment tools not reported
Dolgin et al. (1997) http://dx.doi.org/10.1007/BF02548945	To evaluate effects of structured group intervention for siblings of children with cancer in their cancer-related knowledge, feelings, and attitudes toward childhood cancer and overall mood state.	Level III—Before–after. 23 participants (12 in group with mean age 8.8 years, 11 in group with mean age 13.6 years).	Both child and adolescent intervention included facilitated group discussion, art therapy techniques, role-playing, and informal social interaction. Outcome Measures: Questionnaires on feelings and attitudes, mood and satisfaction, and cancer-related knowledge.	Intervention promoted significant improvements in cancer-related knowledge, facilitated expression of feeling, promoted illness-related communication, and improved mood states for siblings of children with cancer.	No control group Follow-up period limited to 6–8 weeks

Author/Year	Study Objectives	Level/Design/Participants	Intervention and Outcome Measures	Results	Study Limitations
Drysdale et al. (2008)	To evaluate community living skills training and determine its effectiveness for improving the functional ability of children with moderate learning disabilities.	Level I—Blinded randomized controlled trial. N = 40—30 male, 10 female Ages 9–11 years with moderate intellectual disabilities	Participants were assigned to one of three groups, including Treatment Group 1 (classroom and community-based training), Treatment Group 2 (classroom-based), and control (normal classroom activities). The intervention included groups of six children engaging in activities of instruction, demonstration, role play, group exercise, games, and discussion. A range of functional skills also was covered: road safety, money concepts, shopping, preparing snacks, using the telephone, and finding information. Outcome Measures: Task analyses of shopping and telephone tasks.	Community living skills training was effective in improving the functional ability of children with intellectual disabilities in tasks related to shopping. Performance on the shopping task improved for both intervention groups compared to the control group, but there was no difference between the two intervention groups. There was no difference in performance between all three groups on the telephone tasks.	The sample size of each group was small, which limits the validity of the study. Also, only two visits to each shop were completed in community-based sessions, which limits reproducibility. The improvement on the shopping task might have been increased because of the presence of a reinforcer (bought a snack and drink). Researchers used pretend telephone calls, which limits the concreteness of the task. The initial steps in task analysis were more complicated than later ones, which could have limited outcomes.

http://dx.doi.org/10.1080/11038120802456136

Dubow et al. (1987)	To examine effects of cognitive, behavioral, combined cognitive–behavioral, or attention/play training for children identified as clinically aggressive in school.	Level II—Nonrandomized controlled trial. 104 aggressive elementary school boys. Mean age 10.3 years (range 8–13 years).	Participants received cognitive (self-control) training by cue cards and role-playing, behavioral (prosocial skills) training by role-playing, cognitive–behavioral training, and attention/play training with board games and card games. Outcome Measures: • Teacher ratings of aggression and prosocial behavior • Child peer nominations transformed into teacher rating of aggression and prosocial behavior.	Children receiving cognitive–behavioral and attention/play training had a reduction of aggressive behavior and increase of prosocial behavior. At 6-month follow-up, improvement was maintained in attention/play training group.	Lack of random assignment Evaluation of interventions is based solely on teacher rating of children and behavior.

http://dx.doi.org/10.1016/0005-7967(87)90061-1

(Continued)

Table C.2. Targeted Interventions

Author/Year	Study Objectives	Level/Design/Participants	Intervention and Outcome Measures	Results	Study Limitations
Duffy & Fuller (2000) http://dx.doi.org/10.1046/j.1468-3148.2000.00011.x	To examine effectiveness of music and non-music therapy program in enhancement of social skills of children with moderate intellectual disability.	Level I—Randomized controlled trial. 32 children with moderate intellectual disability. Ages 5–10 years. I—Randomized controlled trial. 20 preschool-age children with developmental delay (ages 15–62 months) and their mothers (ages 26–50 years). III—Before–after. 10 adolescents (mean age 16 years) diagnosed with mental retardation or Down syndrome.	All participants randomly assigned to music and non-music therapy programs. Music program promoted social skills by music activities, songs, and music materials. Nonmusic program facilitated social skills without music activities. Outcome Measures: • Social skills test • Occurrences of initiations and vocalizations in pre and posttest • Evaluation questionnaire from staff in posttest.	Both music and non-music programs demonstrated significant improvements on target social skills for children with moderate Intellectual disability.	Reliability and validity for outcome measures not reported
Fantuzzo et al. (1996) http://dx.doi.org/10.1037/0022-006X.64.6.1377	To examine differences in interactive peer play between abused and not abused and socially withdrawn children and effectiveness of resilient peer treatment (RPT).	Level I—Randomized controlled trial. 46 participants: 20 abused or neglected, 26 not abused or neglected (19 boys, 27 girls). Ages 3–5 years.	All participants randomly assigned to RPT in which a play supporter (parent volunteer) allowed target child and resilient peer to play in classroom or dyad played without RPT. Outcome Measures: • Peer play observation • Social skills rating system • Peer play interactive checklist.	RPT facilitated significant increase in positive interactive peer play and decrease in solitary play for abused or neglected or not abused, socially withdrawn children. Effects maintained for 2 months' posttreatment.	No extended period of follow-up. Because all participants were from low-income families, may be difficult to generalize to other populations.
Frankel et al. (1997) http://dx.doi.org/10.1097/00004583-199708000-00013	To evaluate and demonstrate generalization of outpatient social-skills training program when parents are trained in skills relevant to child's social adjustment.	Level II—Nonrandomized controlled trial (wait-list controls). 49 in experimental group, 24 in wait-list controls. Ages 6–12 years. Diagnosis of ADHD and on a stimulant medication or ODD.	Social-skills training intervention included 1-on-1 session, group sessions, coached play, discipline and rewards, and parent sessions and child socialization homework. Outcome Measures: • Structured Diagnostic Interview • Social Skills Rating System • Pupil Evaluation Inventory.	Children with ADHD are best helped by a combination of social-skills training for themselves, collateral training for their parents, and stimulant medication.	Lack of random assignment Groups differed significantly in mean socioeconomic status. No evaluation of peers included

Gebert et al. (1998)	To evaluate if asthma training would give children greater responsibility in everyday asthma self-management.	Level I—Randomized controlled trial. 81 participants with asthma. Ages 7–14 years (mean age 9 years). 27 participants in training group 1, 29 in training group 2, 25 in control group.	Asthma training program of group seminars on training technique, medical model of asthma, social activity, physiotherapy, sport, and relaxation techniques. Training group 1 included asthma training plus 6 monthly follow-up sessions; training group 2 included same training without follow-ups; control group contained guidelines without additional training. Outcome Measures: • Standardized health locus of control and anxiety scales of German personality questionnaire for children • Medical examination • Treadmill stress tests.	A self-management program is effective in improving knowledge about prevention and treatment of asthma for participants. Training Group 1 benefited most with respect to active asthma self-management. Training Group 2 benefited to some degree, whereas control group did not show any benefit.	No long-term analysis of outcome
http://dx.doi.org/10.1016/S0738-3991(98)00061-5					
Gencoz (1997)	To examine the effects of basketball training on maladaptive behaviors of children with mental retardation.	Level I—Randomized controlled trial. 10 in experimental group, 10 in control group. Mean age 12 years (range 10–14 years). Diagnosis of mental retardation.	Experimental group: Participated in 7-week program (Sports Skills Instructional Program) to teach rules of basketball along with sportsmanship and team tactics. Control group: Played with similar balls without any instruction. Outcome Measures: • American Association on Mental Deficiency on Adaptive Behavior Scale • Classroom Behavior Checklist • Sport Skills Assessment.	Children with mental retardation were able to learn not only basic dribbling, shooting, and passing skills, but also regulations of basketball, and they developed sportsmanship. Research also indicated generalization to classroom and home at postassessment and follow-up.	Small sample size
http://dx.doi.org/10.1016/S0891-4222(96)00029-7					

(Continued)

Table C.2. Targeted Interventions

Author/Year	Study Objectives	Level/Design/Participants	Intervention and Outcome Measures	Results	Study Limitations
Girolametto (1988) http://dx.doi.org/10.4061/2011/179124	To examine impact of social–conversational skills program on parents and their children with developmental delay.	Level I—Randomized controlled trial. 20 preschool-age children with developmental delay (ages 15–62 months) and their mothers (ages 26–50 years).	All participants randomly assigned to experimental and control groups. Experimental group (Hanen Early Language Parent Program) included group sessions (observation, following child's lead, play, music) and home visits. Control group received no intervention. Outcome Measures: • Social conversational skills by Griffiths Mental Development Scales • Videotape of parent–child interaction • Sequenced Inventory of Communication Development.	Training parents of children with developmental delay to increase their use of conversation strategies had a positive impact on their children's social–conversational skills.	Small sample size
Guy et al. (2011)	To systematically review the literature on active and educational videogames targeting diet and physical activity in children.	Level I—Systematic review. Review of PubMed and Embase 1998–2011.	Systematic review of 34 studies on exergaming and educational videogames to encourage physical activity and a healthy diet. Outcome measures • Level of physical activity • Playing time • Energy expenditure • Game satisfaction • Servings of fruit and vegetables per day • Nutritional knowledge.	There was increased physical activity and nutritional knowledge following participation in exergaming and educational videogames. Results showed some benefit (increased physical activity and nutritional knowledge as a result of gaming).	Included a variety of studies of healthy and at-risk children Limited number of databases included
Hepler & Rose (1988) http://dx.doi.org/10.1300/J079v11n04_01	To examine effects of multicomponent group approach for improving social skills of elementary school children.	Level II—Before–after with control group. 40 participants included popular students and low-status students. Mean age 10.5 years in treatment group, 10.4 years in control group.	Treatment group (20 participants) consisted of problem-solving techniques, social skills, recreational activities, and small group intervention strategies. Control group (20 participants) received no treatment. Outcome Measures: • Sociometric status by ratings of how well-liked children are by their peers • Social skills by a locus of control test and a role-play test • Pretest, posttest, and 4-week follow-up.	Multicomponent group approach improved social skills for elementary school students. Students in treatment group showed significant improvement on sociometric ratings. Low-status children in treatment group showed significant improvement on negative peer nominations.	Control group not randomized Small sample size for analyzing rejected children Reliability and validity of outcome measures not reported

Study	Purpose	Design/Sample	Intervention and Outcome Measures	Results	Limitations
Hernandez-Guzman et al. (2002)	To evaluate the effectiveness of guided imagery on social behavior of withdrawn and rejected first graders during play.	Level 1—Randomized controlled trial. $N = 40$ withdrawn and rejected first graders in Mexico $n = 8$ in each of 4 conditions plus control.	Interventions: Four guided imagery condition (mastery plus peer acceptance, mastery with no social contingency, coping, and gradual rehearsal). Control: No intervention. Outcome Measure: Behavioral Observation Code – social interactions/behavior during free play at recess.	Positive socialization was observed in mastery plus peer acceptance, mastery with no social contingency, and coping. At follow-up, increased, socialization was maintained only for the coping condition (guided imagery of failure to get peer acceptance, but progressively mastering the social intervention and being accepted by peers).	Small sample sizes Dropouts at follow-up
http://dx.doi.org/10.1017/S1352465802004083					
Jackson & Marzillier (1983)	To examine treatment effects of therapeutic youth club for adolescents with social difficulty.	Level 1—Randomized controlled trial. 16 shy and withdrawn adolescents with social difficulty. Ages 13–16 years (11 boys, 5 girls).	Social-skills training youth club treatment group contained structured social activities. 8 participants in group received social-skills training and youth club activities. 8 were assigned in wait-list control group. Outcome Measures: • Social skills by Social Problem Checklist • Target Ratings • Social Self-Esteem Questionnaire • Social Activities Form • Social Contracts Form • Parents Questionnaire Conversation Test.	There was no difference in social skills outcomes for those participating in social-skills training/Youth Club and those on wait-list.	Small sample size Intervention period may be too short to demonstrate treatment effects. Reliability and validity of the assessments not reported
http://dx.doi.org/10.1017/S0141347300008612					
Jeffree & Cheseldine (1984)	To determine whether interaction with peers would increase and if higher level of activity would result if specific leisure skills were taught to teenagers with severe mental retardation.	Level III—Before–after. 10 adolescents (mean age 16 years) diagnosed with mental retardation or Down syndrome.	In preintervention session, leisure activities (e.g, board and construction games, puzzles, card games) were introduced to group. At 2-week intervention, new games were introduced at increasingly more difficult level. Participants then introduced to peer who could play at that level. Outcome Measure: Observation of interaction (solitary, interactive–adult, interactive–peer).	After treatment, participants with mental retardation showed higher levels of interaction with their peers when involved in more skilled activities.	Small sample size Lack of a control group Short intervention period to reveal effect of treatment

(Continued)

Table C.2. Targeted Interventions

Author/Year	Study Objectives	Level/Design/Participants	Intervention and Outcome Measures	Results	Study Limitations
Kamps et al. (2000)	To examine effects of 2-year prevention program on social skills and behavior for children with behavioral problems.	Level I—Randomized controlled trial. 31 participants in experimental group—19 in Cohort 1, 12 in Cohort 2, 18 in comparison group. Mean age for experimental group = 60.9 months; mean age for control group = 57 months.	Both cohorts received 2 years of social skills intervention that included toys, board games, and special projects. Parent support intervention included group activities. Control group received no treatment. Outcome Measures: • Direct observation of student classroom behavior • Teacher ratings • Direct observation of peer interaction using Multi-Option Observation System for Experimental Studies code.	Participants who received social interventions indicated higher levels of peer interaction and fewer inappropriate behaviors in their classrooms than students in comparison group.	Small sample size Lack of outcome measure from parent reports Variation in participation rates of participants during 2-year intervention period Potential insensitivity of assessment instrument of teachers' ratings of students' classroom behaviors
Kazdin et al. (1989) http://dx.doi.org/10.1037/0022-006X.57.4.522	To examine effects of cognitive–behavioral therapy and relationship therapy for reducing behavior problems and improving functioning at home and at school for children with antisocial behaviors.	Level I—Randomized controlled trial. 112 participants with antisocial behaviors in pretest, 97 remained in posttest, and 93 remained in follow-up. Mean age 11 years (range 7–13 years).	Children randomly assigned to problem-solving skills training, problem-solving skills training within vivo practice, and client-centered relationship therapy. Outcome Measures: Antisocial behaviors; prosocial behaviors at home and school.	Children in problem-solving skills training and problem-solving skills training with in vivo practice showed significantly greater reductions in antisocial behavior and overall behavior problems and greater increases in prosocial behavior than those in client-centered relationship therapy.	Did not assess cognitive processes that problem-solving skills training were designed to change. Did not reflect which treatment worked with specific participants under different conditions.
Kingsnorth et al. (2007) http://dx.doi.org/10.1016/j.jadohealth.2007.06.007	To evaluate the effectiveness of life skills programs that emphasize independent functioning in preparation for adulthood for adolescents and young adults with physical disabilities.	Level I—Systematic review. Studies with a comparison group published between 1985–2006 evaluating life skills programs for youth 14–21 years of age.	Interventions: Focused on financial management, meal preparation, and navigation in the community and incorporated problem solving, decision making, goal setting, and skills for coping with stress. Outcome Measures: • Canadian Occupational Performance Measure • Self-image • Self-efficacy • Social Skills Rating System • Role Play Test.	All 6 studies included in the review used a multicomponent group intervention incorporating a real-world or role-play experiential component. 5 of the 6 studies reported short-term improvements in targeted life skills.	Only 2 of 6 studies were randomized controlled trials. Heterogeneity of outcome measures Small sample sizes Studies were heterogeneous for physical disability type.

Lamb et al. (1997) http://dx.doi.org/10.1177/026569097013000304	To examine effects of supported peer communication activities program on communication skills for children with moderate learning difficulties.	Level III—Before–after without control group. 30 participants with moderate learning difficulty. 19 boys, 11 girls. Mean age 14 years.	10 communication activities (dynamic, static, collaborative tasks) used to facilitate communication skills for participants. Outcome Measure: Communication skills by map task used to elicit spontaneous dialogue between pairs of children.	After peer communication activities programs, participants talked more, responded to ambiguous instructions more effectively, and asked more appropriate types of questions. Program was successful in teaching children strategies for handling ambiguities in communication.	No control group Coders not blind to study goal
Lochman et al. (1981) http://dx.doi.org/10.1007/BF00706674	To examine psychosocial effects of intensive summer communication program for children with cleft lip and palate.	Level III—Before–after without control group. 12 children with cleft lip and palate; 8 boys, 4 girls. Mean age 7 years 1 month.	Intensive summer residential program included individual speech–language therapy, psychosocial discussion groups, arts and crafts, music, physical education, field trips, and free play. Outcome Measures: Social interaction by Social Interaction Recording System, Children's Expectancies Parent Form.	Intensive summer program had positive effects on social interaction and expectancies for social interactions with peers (as measured at completion of summer program).	Small sample size No control group No long-term follow-up of outcome
Lochman & Wells (2002) http://dx.doi.org/10.1037/0893-164X.16.4S.S40	To evaluate the effectiveness of Coping Power, a prevention intervention to reduce aggressive and disruptive behaviors in middle school children.	Level I—Randomized controlled trial. $N = 245$ fifth-grade boys identified as aggressive $n = 61$ universal classroom intervention + indicated intervention (IU) $n = 62$ universal classroom intervention + control intervention (U) $n = 59$ universal classroom comparison + indicated intervention (I) $n = 63$ universal classroom comparison + control intervention (C)	Interventions: Universal classroom interventions—parent meetings and teacher in-service for transition to middle school. Indicated Intervention: Coping Power—group sessions focused on problem solving, coping with anxiety and arousal, improving social skills, coping and peer pressure. Outcome Measures: • Proactive–Reactive Aggressive Behavior Scale • Early Adolescent Temperament Measure • Teacher Rating of Children's Social Skill, Perceived Competence Scale for Children.	All 3 intervention cells produced relatively lower rates of substance use at postintervention than did the control cell. The interventions also produced effects on 3 of the 4 predictor variable domains: children's social competence, self-regulation, and parents' parenting skills.	Relatively small sample size Limited to boys

(Continued)

Table C.2. Targeted Interventions

Author/Year	Study Objectives	Level/Design/Participants	Intervention and Outcome Measures	Results	Study Limitations
Lochman & Wells (2003)	To evaluate the 1-year outcomes of above study of Coping Power intervention.	Level I—Randomized controlled trial. As above.	As above.	The Coping Power program, in conjunction with the classroom-level intervention, also reduced school aggression 1 year after the intervention was completed. In addition, it appears that the classroom intervention facilitates radiating effects on reduced substance use for other at-risk children in the same classrooms who did not receive Coping Power.	Relatively small sample size Limited to boys
http://dx.doi.org/10.1016/S0005-7894(03)80032-1					
Lochman & Wells (2004)	To evaluate the 1-year outcomes of above study of Coping Power intervention.	Level I—Randomized controlled trial. As above.	As above.	At 1-year follow-up, participants in Coping Power with parent and child components were less likely to participate in covert delinquent behavior such as theft and property damage. There was no difference for overt delinquency, such as assault or robbery. Teacher-rated behavior improvements were noted in the follow-up year for those in the Coping Power program.	Relatively small sample size Limited to boys
http://dx.doi.org/10.1037/0022-006X.72.4.571					
Lowenstein (1982)	To examine effects of combined treatment, including implosive, counseling, and behavioral approaches on timidity in children with extreme shyness.	Level I—Randomized controlled trial. 11 participants in experimental group, 11 in control group. 16 boys, 6 girls with extreme shyness. Ages 9–16 years.	Experimental group of implosive approaches (including participation in swimming, games, drama therapy), counseling therapy, and behavior therapy. Participants in control group informally encouraged to increase social contact and communication. Outcome Measures: • Timidity and extraversion by Maudsley Personality Inventory • Rating scales of reading, spelling, and mathematic attainment in pretest and posttest.	Children in experimental group showed decreased timidity and increased extraversion compared to control group.	Small sample size Reliability and validity of outcome measures not reported
http://dx.doi.org/10.1111/j.1600-0447.1982.tb00926.x					

Author (Year)	Purpose	Design/Sample	Intervention/Outcome Measures	Results	Limitations
McPherson et al. (2006) http://dx.doi.org/10.1542/peds.2005-0666	To evaluate the effectiveness and acceptability of an educational multimedia program to promote self-management skills in children with asthma.	Level I—Randomized controlled trial. $N = 101$ children age 7–14 under the care of hospital-based asthma services in the United Kingdom. $n = 50$ asthma information booklet + Asthma Files—interactive CD-ROM. $n = 51$ asthma information booklet.	Intervention: Asthma Files is an interactive computer game with a secret agent theme to find out about asthma and self-management. Asthma information booklet was given to both intervention and control groups. Outcome Measures: • Asthma knowledge • Asthma locus of control, school absence.	At 1-month follow-up, children in the Asthma Files group had improved knowledge and a more internal locus of control than the control group. At 6-month follow-up, fewer children in the intervention group had taken time off from school for asthma in the past 6 months than the control group.	No measures of child behavior Researcher not blind to allocation at follow-up
Mevarech & Kramarski (1993) http://dx.doi.org/10.1111/j.2044-8279.1993.tb01044.x	To examine effects of a peer-pairing approach on social interaction and sociometric status for peer-neglected children.	Level II—Nonrandomized controlled trial. 83 8th graders; 43 boys, 40 girls. Mean age 13 years 7.1 months.	Participants studied in 3 classrooms: cooperative Logo environment ($n = 30$), individualized Logo environment ($n = 24$), and non-treatment control group ($n = 29$). Students in Logo-Stat program taught descriptive statistics via Logo and SOLVE strategy (systematic analysis) with or without peers. Outcome Measures: • Creativity and interpersonal relationships by Porteus Maze Test • Torrance Test of Creative Thinking Interpersonal Relations • Assessment Technique.	Students in cooperative Logo environment outperformed their counterparts on certain measures of creativity and developed more positive interpersonal relationships than students in other 2 settings.	Lack of random assignment
Moody et al. (2003)	To evaluate the effectiveness of Youth Empowerment and Support Program (YES-P) to decrease drug use and strengthen school connections in at-risk youth.	Level III—Pretest–posttest design. $N = 13$ children ages 10–12 in an inner-city neighborhood with a history of one or more of the following: exposure to violence, family history of substance abuse or mental illness, abuse or neglect, involvement in juvenile crime.	Intervention: The YES-P is an activity- and community-based program incorporating mentor support, social skills training, forming a positive peer culture, and developing youth in leadership roles for community service. Outcome Measure: Questions regarding self-esteem, school bonding, social skills, attitudes toward drugs.	Percentage change was highest for group bonding, social skills, and self-esteem. Attitudes against underage drug use decreased from pretest scores.	Small sample size Limited validity of evaluation measure

(Continued)

Table C.2. Targeted Interventions

Author/Year	Study Objectives	Level/Design/Participants	Intervention and Outcome Measures	Results	Study Limitations
Morris et al. (1995)	To examine effects of cooperative and individualized Logo environments on creativity and interpersonal relationships regarding academic recognition and social acceptance.	Level I—Randomized controlled trial. 72 1st and 2nd graders (24 peer-neglected, 24 popular, 24 average children). 36 boys, 36 girls.	Peer-neglected and popular children randomly assigned to conditions. In treatment group, each neglected child paired with same-sex popular child. Pairs engaged in series of joint-task activities requiring interaction. Outcome Measures: • Social interaction and sociometric status by sociometrics (degree a child is liked by his or her peer group) • Playground observations (positive and negative interaction, solitary play).	Peer-pairing intervention for neglected children resulted in dramatic improvement in social status and social interaction. Improvements remained stable through 1-month follow-up assessment.	Whether peer-pairing intervention or classroom activities facilitated social interaction and sociometric status unknown.
http://dx.doi.org/10.1207/s1537442jccp2401_2					
O'Connor et al. (2007)	To evaluate the effectiveness of a social-skills training program for children with fetal alcohol syndrome (FAS).	Level II—Nonrandomized controlled trial. N = 100 children 6–12 years of age with FAS n = 49 children, friendship training (CFT) n = 51 children, delayed treatment control (DTC)	Interventions: CFT—social skills training previously validated empirically in multiple clinical contexts. CFT includes modeling, feedback, rehearsal, and homework. Control: DTC. Outcome Measures: • Test of Social Skills Knowledge • Social Skills Rating System.	Children in the CFT group had significantly more improvement in knowledge of appropriate social behavior, and according to parent report, compared to DTC. CFT resulted in improved social skills and fewer problem behaviors compared with DTC. Gains were maintained at 3-month follow-up. After receiving treatment, the DTC group exhibited similar improvement. Teachers did not report improvement as a function of social-skills treatment.	Study limited to participants with IQ of 70 and above
http://dx.doi.org/10.1037/0022-006X.74.4.639					
Ohl et al. (2008)	To evaluate the effectiveness of the Pyramid Club on children's social–emotional health.	Level II—Nonrandomized controlled trial. N = 105 Year 3 primary school children in London n = 43 Pyramid Club (children identified as a cause for concern) n = 62 nonproblem comparison.	Interventions: The Pyramid Club is a 10-week group program in an after-school club that focuses on building confidence, well-being, and friendship skills. Control: Nonproblem comparison Outcome Measure: Goodman Strengths and Difficulties Questionnaire (SDQ).	Postintervention both groups had improved Total Difficulty scores on SDQ, with the Pyramid Club group showing a significantly stronger effect size than the nonproblem comparison group.	Follow-up only at end of intervention Use of a nonproblem comparison group
http://dx.doi.org/10.1111/j.1475-3588.2007.00476.x					

Citation	Study Design/Participants	Intervention/Outcome Measures	Results	Limitations
Powell et al. (2008)	To evaluate the effectiveness of a combined massage, yoga, and relaxation program for children receiving special education and those with emotional and behavioral difficulties.	Level II—Nonrandomized controlled trial. N = 107 children ages 8–11 years in special education classes and with behavioral and emotional difficulties at risk of being asked to leave school. n = 53 intervention n = 54 control	Intervention: Self-discovery program that included massage, yoga, breathwork, and relaxation. Control: Did not participate in program. Outcome Measures: • Behavioral profiles—self and social confidence • Communication abilities • Self-control • Attention span • Strengths and difficulties questionnaire.	Participants in the intervention group showed improvements in self-confidence, social confidence, communication, and contribution in class compared to the control group. Teachers reported that children in intervention group used learned skills during the school day.	Lack of randomization Difference between groups may represent increased attention to intervention group.

http://dx.doi.org/10.1080/08856250802387398

Citation	Study Design/Participants	Intervention/Outcome Measures	Results	Limitations
Rickel et al. (1983)	To evaluate effectiveness of Spivack and Shure training program in facilitating long-term and durable changes in cognitive interpersonal problem-solving skills and behavior adjustment for young children.	Level II—Nonrandomized controlled trial. 37 participants with aberrant defects or adjusted defects. Ages 4 years 9 months–5 years 9 months.	Spivack and Shure program of series of brief, primarily verbal, daily games involving small groups of 4–6 children. Games dealt with understanding of selected language skills, likes and dislikes of children, and concept of fairness. Final lessons of series of real-life problems that involved a synthesis of skills and concepts learned in program. Outcome Measures: • Cognitive interpersonal problem solving skills • Behavioral adjustment.	Children in social problem-solving group gained significantly compared to controls in cognitive abilities to generate alternative solutions to interpersonal problems at posttest, but this effect was not found at follow-up. No significant behavioral training effects were revealed at posttest or follow-up.	Lack of random assignment Normal maturational processes and general educational stimulation could improve alternative solutions, consequential thinking, and achievement.

http://dx.doi.org/10.1007/BF00912174

Citation	Study Design/Participants	Intervention/Outcome Measures	Results	Limitations
Robertson & Weistmer (1997)	To investigate influence of peer models on play scripts of children with specific language impairment (SLI).	Level I—Randomized controlled trial. 20 participants with specific language impairment (mean age 4 years 2 months) and 10 with normal language abilities (mean age 4 years 4 months).	Children with SLI randomly assigned to experimental (SLI-E) group or control (SLI-C) group. SLI-E group had 4 dyadic play sessions with different peer models. SLI-C group had same play props as SLI-E group without peer models. Outcome Measures: • Number of words (productivity), different words, and play-theme related acts • Linguistic markers by scripts of playing house.	Children in SLI-E group improved their number of word use, number of different words, number of play-theme-related acts, and use of linguistic markers in their play scripts after treatment compared to those in SLI-C group.	Small sample size

(Continued)

Table C.2. Targeted Interventions

Author/Year	Study Objectives	Level/Design/Participants	Intervention and Outcome Measures	Results	Study Limitations
Santomier & Kopczuk (1981)	To examine effects of teacher intervention (pairing student with trainable mental retardation [TMR] with nonretarded students) and verbal reinforcement on social interaction for students with TMR in integrated physical education program.	Level I—Randomized controlled trial. 6 in experimental group 1, 6 in experimental group 2, 6 in control group. Mean age 13 years. Trainable mental retardation.	Experimental group 1: Program of teacher-directed physical activities, teacher intervention (pairing TMR with nonretarded students), and teacher praise for motor skill performance. Experimental group 2: Program of teacher-directed physical activities, teacher intervention (pairing TMR with nonretarded students), and teacher praise for social interaction. Control group: Program of teacher directed physical activities and teacher praise for motor skill performance. Outcome Measure: Videotaping and observing number and type of social interactions.	Students in experimental group 2 consistently had higher total interaction rates, social interaction rates between TMR and nonretarded students, and cooperative social interaction rates than those in experimental group 1 or control group.	Small sample size Blinding of experimenters not reported Posttest period limited to 3 weeks
Schery & O'Connor (1992)	To examine effect of computer-based language intervention on communication skills for children with multiple physical and mental disabilities.	Level II—Nonrandomized controlled trial. 52 participants with multiple severe impairments. Mean age 5.9 years (3.3–12.9 years).	Programs for Early Acquisition of Language software, including Exploratory Play and Representational Play, used in treatment. In programs, computer-vocalized vocabulary as graphic was displayed, and a graduate student interacted with participant to match and then display real objects. Outcome Measures: Vocabulary, language, and social/interpersonal skills.	Computer training improved trained vocabulary, general language skills, and social/interpersonal functioning of all participants with multiple severe disabilities.	Reliability and validity of outcome measures not reported No clear descriptions of how outcomes were assessed Treatment effect on different genders and diagnoses unknown
Shechtman (2000) http://dx.doi.org/10.1002/(SICT)1520-6807 (20003)37:2<157::AID-PITS7>3.0.CO:2-G	To evaluate effectiveness of an intervention to reduce aggressive behavior among children and adolescents.	Level I—Randomized controlled trial. 70 participants: 34 in treatment group (29 boys, 5 girls), 36 in control group (26 boys, 10 girls). All participants from special education classroom. Ages 10–15 years.	Bibliotherapy program including short stories, poems, and films provided to treatment group. Literacy pieces carefully selected to include themes of aggression. Outcome Measures: Child Behavior Checklist, teacher report form regarding students' behavior.	Structured activity-based bibliotherapy program was more effective than control intervention in reducing aggression and enhancing well-being in a special education population.	Long-term effect not shown 3 types of interventions not compared (individual, pairs, and small groups)

Study	Level/Design/Participants	Intervention and Outcome Measures	Results	Limitations
Sparling et al. (1984)	To examine effect of educational play and educational drama as intervention approaches for children with neurological impairments.	All children and adults participated in educational drama (ED) and educational art (EA). EA was a medium to stimulate different cognitive levels of subjects. ED included activities with both conflict essential to dramatic experience and duality inherent in pretend or symbolic play. Outcome Measures: • Vulpe Assessment Battery assessed gross and fine motor, language, cognition, ADL, and social–emotional development • Art/drama questionnaire.	Educational play and educational drama could improve gross and fine motor, language, cognition, ADL, and social–emotional development for children with neurological impairments. Participating adults began to value use of play as an essential component of child development.	Lack of control group Limitations of staff prevented pretest and posttest with full Vulpe Assessment Battery rather than selected items.
	Level III—Before–after without control group. 14 children with neurological impairments (9 boys, 5 girls), 18 adults. Mean age of children 4.55 years.			
http://dx.doi.org/10.5014/ajot.38.9.603				
Sussman (2009)	To determine the effect of music on peer awareness in preschool children with developmental disabilities.	Interventions: Music or play group with 4 interventions 1. Music during passing, pass musical object; 2. Music during passing, pass nonmusical object; 3. No music during passing, pass musical object 4. No music during passing, pass nonmusical object Outcome Measures: • Sustained attention • Alternating attention.	Children sustained attention toward peers for the longest durations and alternated attention from peer to peer at the highest frequencies during activities that utilized a musical object within a nonmusical or play-based context.	Small sample size No specific comparison group
	Level II—Within-subject repeated-measures design with children serving as own control. $N = 9$ children ages 2–6 with diagnosis of developmental disability.			
http://dx.doi.org/10.1037/h008943				
Tyndall-Lynd et al. (2001)	To determine effectiveness of psychodynamic play therapy combined with adult-facilitated recreational play and educational experiences with sibling dyads and to compare this to effectiveness of psychodynamic play therapy with individual children and to no intervention.	Child-directed play therapy combined with recreational/educational activities and performed with sibling dyads. Outcome Measures: • Children's behavior by Achenbach Child Behavior Checklist • Joseph Pre-School Primary Self-Concept Screening Test.	Children in experimental group exhibited significant reduction in total behavior problems, externalizing and internalizing behavior problems, aggression, anxiety, and depression, and a significant improvement in self-esteem. Intensive sibling group play therapy was equally effective as intensive individual play therapy with child witnesses of domestic violence.	Small, nonrandomized subject sample Comparison and control groups from different study, which was performed by researchers other than those in this study. Child-directed play therapy intervention mixed with more adult-directed educational and recreational activities during experimental phase, resulting in multiple interventions.
	Level II—Nonrandomized controlled trial. 32 participants from a shelter for victims of domestic violence. 10 in experimental group (mean age 6.2 years), 11 in comparison group (mean age 6.9 years), 11 in control group (mean age 5.9 years).			
http://dx.doi.org/10.1037/h008943				(Continued)

Table C.2. Targeted Interventions

Author/Year	Study Objectives	Level/Design/Participants	Intervention and Outcome Measures	Results	Study Limitations
Udwin (1983)	To examine imaginative play training as intervention method with institutionalized preschool children.	Level I—Randomized controlled trial. 17 institutionalized pre-school children in treatment group, 17 in control group. 10 boys, 7 girls in each group. Mean age 56 months (36–74 months).	In treatment group, imaginative play that consisted of sensory awareness exercises and play with puppets, story reading, and plots design around given themes. Control children engaged in construction-type play with blocks and puzzles. Outcome Measures: • Assessment of imaginative play, Guilford Unusual Used Test • Children's Apperception Test, Wechsler Pre-School and Primary Intelligence • Goodenough Draw-a-Man Test.	When compared to matched controls, experimental group showed significant increments on levels of imaginative play, positive emotional feelings, and prosocial behavior, and in measures of divergent thinking and storytelling skills. Decreases in levels of overt aggression were also shown.	No follow-up assessment

http://dx.doi.org/10.1111/j.2044-8279.1983.tb02533.x

Author/Year	Study Objectives	Level/Design/Participants	Intervention and Outcome Measures	Results	Study Limitations
Waddell et al. (2007)	To examine the effectiveness of interventions to prevent conduct disorder (CD), anxiety, and depression in children ages 0–18.	Level I—Systematic review of RCTs. Databases searched: MEDLINE, PsycINFO, Cochrane Database from 1981–2003.	Interventions to prevent CD, anxiety, and depression, primarily targeted for at-risk children, with 2 universal programs included. Interventions include social skills training (SST), parent training (PT), and cognitive–behavioral training (CBT). Outcome Measures: • Child Behavior Checklist • Eyberg Child Behavior Inventory • Social Behavior Questionnaire • Teacher and parent ratings.	Thirty articles on 15 RCTs met the criteria. Ten demonstrated significant reductions in child symptom and/or diagnostic measures at follow-up. For CD, the strongest targeted at-risk children in the early years using PT or SST; for anxiety, universal CBT in school-age children; and depression, targeted at-risk school-age children using CBT.	Some studies included in the review were limited by lack of blinding and failure to designate and report primary outcomes at all time points.
Wade et al. (2006)	To examine whether an online cognitive–behavioral intervention could improve child adjustment following traumatic brain injury (TBI).	Level I—Randomized controlled trial. N = 40 families of 5- to 16-year-old children with moderate to severe TBI. n = 20 family problem-solving group (FPS) n = 20 Internet resources comparison (IRC)	Interventions: Both groups received psychosocial care, computer, printer. FPS received a 14-session Web-based online problem-solving skills training with exercises plus videoconference with therapist. IRC: Access to home page of brain injury resources and links. Outcome Measures: • Child Behavior Checklist • Socioeconomic status (SES).	The FPS group reported better child self-management/compliance at follow-up than did the IRC group. The child's age and SES moderated treatment effects, with older children and those of lower SES who received FPS showing greater improvements in self-management and behavior problems, respectively.	Small sample size Sample skewed to those with less severe injury A higher proportion of the IRC group received group therapy than those in FPS group.

| Walsh et al. (1991) | To examine effects of 2 school-based, short-term creative drama programs in small groups on peer interaction skills for children and early adolescents with social–emotional and cognitive difficulties. | Level II—Nonrandomized controlled trial.

Study I
12 7th graders in fall group and 9 in winter group (delay treatment).
All participants had social–emotional and cognitive difficulties.
Study II
15 participants with peer problems in treatment group (7 in younger group and 8 in older group) and 9 in comparison group.
Ages 9–12 years in older group and 6–9 years in younger group. | *Study I*
Drama activity allowed participants to choose their own storylines and characters, play their roles with conviction, self-reflect, and provide constructive criticism to others about their performance. Children's self-efficacy for peer interaction scale by students, Child Behavior Rating Scale (CBRS) by teachers, and parent evaluation of CBRS by parents.
Study II
Same drama programs as in Study I were used in younger and older groups, and results compared to untreated students.

Outcome Measures:
• Children's self-efficacy for peer interaction scale by students
• Group participation scale by parents and teachers
• Inventory of personal, social, and learning skills. | *Study I*
Though there were no quantitative differences for treatment and control groups, participants reported feeling more self-confident about handling peer conflict after the treatment period.
Study II
Experimental group significantly exceeded comparison group on gains in self-confidence in handling peer conflict and on teacher ratings of social–emotional skills. | Small sample size
Rater expectancy effects and random assignment of treatment and comparison groups hard to control.
Intervention period might not be long enough to indicate treatment effects. |
| Wiener & Harris (1997) | To estimate effectiveness of individualized context based social-skills training program for children with learning disabilities. | Level I—Randomized controlled trial.

Total number 45, 8–12 years. 13 in intervention 1, 7 in intervention 2, 25 in control group.
Randomized by class—children with learning disabilities. | Intervention 1: 6-week social-skills training program (SST) and 6-week academic-skills training (AST). Intervention 2: 12-week SST program. Control group: No treatment, but only 19 did not receive SST, AST, or any social-skills training.

Outcome Measures:
• Classroom and playground observations
• Social Skills Rating System (Teacher and Student)
• Child Behavior Checklist
• Self-Perception Profile for Learning Disabled Students
• Peer nominations. | Participants in intervention group 1 had improved social skills and decreased problem behaviors compared to control group. Peer acceptance of intervention group 1 children remained stable over school year. Equivalent changes were not observed in intervention group 2. | Participants in intervention group 2 may have had a learning disability combined with ADHD or conduct disorder, which may have influenced treatment results. |

(Continued)

Table C.2. Targeted Interventions

Author/Year	Study Objectives	Level/Design/Participants	Intervention and Outcome Measures	Results	Study Limitations
Wilfey et al. (2007)	To evaluate the efficacy of lifestyle interventions to reduce childhood overweight.	Level I—Meta-analysis. MEDLINE, PsycINFO, and Cochrane Controlled Trials Register. Searched from first available year to 2005.	RCTs that evaluated weight loss or weight control programs for youth 19 years and younger. Diet, exercise, parental involvement, and self-monitoring were among interventions included. Fourteen RCTs were available. Outcome measures include: • Percentage overweight • z-body mass index (BMI) • BMI • Weight.	Lifestyle interventions yielded significant treatment effects compared to no treatment/ wait-list and information/ education-only control groups. These effects were found both immediately following treatment and at follow-up.	Patient study features (e.g., ethnicity, socioeconomic status) were infrequently reported in included studies.

http://dx.doi.org/10.1037/0278-6133.26.5.521

Note. ADHD = attention deficit hyperactivity disorder; ODD = oppositional defiant disorder; ADL = activities of daily living; RCT = randomized controlled trial.

Table C.3. Intensive Interventions

Author/Year	Study Objectives	Level/Design/Participants	Intervention and Outcome Measures	Results	Study Limitations
Aldred et al. (2004)	To evaluate a theoretically based social communication intervention targeting parental communication for children with autism.	Level I—Randomized controlled trial. 28 children with autism between the ages of 2 years and 5 years, 11 months old. $n = 14$ intervention $n = 14$ control	Interventions: The program followed a developmental progression of early prelinguistic skill (e.g., joint attention) and established a communication environment with parents. After initial training, parents had monthly sessions for 6 months, with less frequent after. Control: Usual care. Outcome Measures: • Autism Diagnostic Observation Schedule (ADOS) • Vineland Adaptive Behavior Scale (VABS) • MacArthur Communicative Developmental Inventory (MCDI) • Parenting Stress Index (PSI) • Parent–child interaction.	Children in the active treatment group showed significantly greater effects on the ADOS than control group. Treatment group made significant gains in areas of expressive language skills as measured by the MCDI. Increased adaptive behavior scores on the VABS were noted in both groups. The parent–child interaction video code showed significant increases in positive synchronous communication and child communication. The PSI reported no difference in parents' stress level from pre- to posttest.	Limited description of intervention strategies Small sample size
			http://dx.doi.org/10.1111/j.1469-7610.2004.00338.x		
Amish et al. (1988)	To evaluate use of traditional cognitive problem-solving methods integrated with behavioral teaching methods of social-skills literature with severely emotionally disturbed children.	Level II—Nonrandomized control trial. 25 in experimental group, 25 in control group. Ages 7–12 years (mean age 9.5 years). Diagnosis of conduct disorder, ADD, oppositional disorder, and adjustment disorder.	Intervention consisted of 15 highly structured classroom-based lessons that taught a systematic approach to solving interpersonal problems. Lessons were presented using competitive games, role-play, videotape, modeling, and feedback. Outcome Measures: • Structure interview (Open Middle Interview) • Role-play assessment • Simulating Problem Solving (SIMPS) • Classroom Rating Scale • Health Resource Inventory • Sociometric rating.	Experimental group generated significantly more alternatives and prosocial alternatives in role-play situations than control group. No differences were noted in adjustment measures and relationships between problems.	Lack of randomization Although SIMPS was originally designed as a posttest measure, it was used here pre- and posttest.

(Continued)

Table C.3. Intensive Interventions

Author/Year	Study Objectives	Level/Design/Participants	Intervention and Outcome Measures	Results	Study Limitations
Baker et al. (2009) http://dx.doi.org/10.1353/etc.0.0065	To systematically review the effectiveness of video modeling as an intervention for students with emotional and behavioral disorders (EBDs) to increase peer interactions and on-task behavior as well as decrease inappropriate behaviors to participate in productive tasks and comply with adult directives.	Level I—Systematic review of 16 studies. Included 93 participants with EBDs.	Description: Video modeling: Individual watched a video of him- or herself engaging in the targeted behavior for improvement. Some studies included in the review used a combination of video modeling plus discussion or other intervention methods. Outcome Measures: Although outcome measures are not reported, the following outcomes were examined: appropriate/inappropriate interactions, on-task behaviors, appropriate/inappropriate/cooperative behaviors, and fidgeting.	Participants demonstrated desired skills in relevant settings, and all showed improvement in varying degrees (increasing peer interaction, increasing on-task behavior, and decreasing inappropriate behavior). Intervention demonstrated the ability to strengthen participants' beliefs in their capabilities. The video modeling actively involved students in a process of self-evaluation and enhanced their ability to accept responsibility for their actions.	The video modeling practices in this study were part of a package, which limits the sole effectiveness of video modeling. The feasibility and suitability of the intervention were not measured consistently across all studies. All studies also did not include the ethnicity of participants. Most of the studies were conducted in special education classrooms or residential facilities, which may not be considered the least restrictive environment.
Bauminger (2007) http://dx.doi.org/10.1007/s10803-006-0245-4	To examine the effects of a social-skills training program with children who have high-functioning autism spectrum disorder (HFASD).	Level III—Pretest–posttest study. $N = 19$ children (18 M, 1 F) between 7 years, 7 months and 11 years, 6 months; 10 with HFASD, 9 with Asperger syndrome). Observers and data collectors were blinded to hypotheses and goals but were not blinded to treatment status.	Intervention: A multimodal cognitive–behavioral ecological (CB-E) social-skills training program that enhances social problem solving, emotional knowledge and recognition, and social interaction abilities using individual treatment. The first year of this study was dedicated to individual training. Outcome Measures: • The Companionship Measure was used to assess the child's ability to interact efficiently in peer groups • Social Interaction Observation Scale • The Problem Solving Measure.	At posttest, children were more likely to initiate interaction and respond positively to peers, especially in eye contact and sharing; in social communication, children were more likely to initiate than to respond. Significant improvement in 3 areas of social skills (cooperation, assertion, and self-control) was found from pre- to posttest. After treatment, significantly more relevant and less passive solutions were found in the children with HFASD.	Lack of a control group For both groups in the two part study, medications and other therapies were not reported. Interventions took place at each child's own school, so other settings have not been tested. Teachers were familiar to children, so unfamiliar teachers also have not been tested.
Butler et al. (2006) http://dx.doi.org/10.1016/j.cpr.2005.07.003	To review the meta-analysis literature on treatment outcomes of cognitive–behavioral therapy (CBT) on a range of psychiatric disorders.	Level I—Systematic review of meta-analyses. PsycINFO, ERIC, and MEDLINE were searched.	16 meta-analyses that included collectively 9,995 subjects in 332 studies. These meta-analyses included 562 comparisons covering 16 childhood, adolescent, and adult disorders. Outcome Measures: Effect sizes of individual meta-analyses.	The authors found large effect sizes when CBT was used for childhood depressive and anxiety disorders. Effect sizes for childhood somatic disorders were moderate.	Aggregation of effect sizes in meta-analyses may mask important variability among studies in methodological rigor, sample characteristics, and measurement instruments.

Cook et al. (2008)	To evaluate the effectiveness of social-skills training (SST) for secondary students with emotion and/or behavioral disorders (EBDs).	Level I—Meta-analyses. Excluded meta-analyses of single-subject design studies. Searched MEDLINE, Psyc-INFO, and ERIC. Although 5 meta-analyses were included in the review and included 367 studies, only 77 that studied adolescents were in the analysis.	Outcome Measure: Social skills performance.	There was a medium effect size for SST, with improvements in two-thirds of secondary students with EBD compared to one-third of controls. Effect sizes were strongest for operant procedures, modeling, and social-cognitive procedures.	Although the authors reported using a descriptive approach, there are no standards for a meta-analysis of meta-analyses.
http://dx.doi.org/10.1177/1063426608314541					
Dobson et al. (1995)	To compare effectiveness of social-skills training and a social-milieu support approach in reducing symptoms of schizophrenia.	Level I—Randomized controlled trial. 33 began study, 15 completed social-skills training, 13 completed social milieu treatment. Ages 18–55 years. Diagnosis of schizophrenia.	Social-skills group met for 4 1-hour sessions over 9 weeks and used direct instruction, communication games, role-playing, modeling, feedback, and daily homework. Social-milieu group had choice of structured activities, including supportive discussion, exercise, and activity groups. Outcome Measures: • Positive and Negative Syndrome Scale • Structured Clinical Interview for DSM–III–R, measuring both positive and negative symptoms of schizophrenia and general psychopathology.	Both treatments were effective in reducing symptoms, but social-skills training appeared to be more effective in reducing negative symptoms. No differences were found between treatment groups in relapse rates or in symptom measures at 3-month follow up. However, 6-month follow-up available only for social-skills training group showed that improvement in negative symptoms had begun to decline.	Small sample size Long-term follow-up only done for social-skills group
Epp (2008)	To evaluate the effectiveness of a social-skills program using art and group therapy for children and adolescents on the autism spectrum.	Level III—Pretest–posttest design. $N = 66$ 11- to 18-year-olds on the autism spectrum enrolled at social-skills program.	Intervention: The SuperKids program is a group therapy program incorporating cognitive–behavioral techniques using art activities and games to improve social skills such as compromise, conversation and friendship skill, and eye contact. Outcome Measure: Social Skills Rating System.	Results indicated a significant improvement in assertion scores, coupled with decreased internalizing behaviors, hyperactivity scores, and problem behavior scores in the students.	Lack of control group Participants were from a primarily affluent community, limiting generalizability.
http://dx.doi.org/10.1093/cs/30.1.27					

(Continued)

Table C.3. Intensive Interventions

Author/Year	Study Objectives	Level/Design/Participants	Intervention and Outcome Measures	Results	Study Limitations
Gangl (1987)	To investigate effects of occupational therapy (work and relationship skills group) on behavioral change of adolescents with chemical dependence and emotional disturbance.	Level III—Before–after. 33 adolescents ages 13–17 years in a residential treatment center with a diagnosis of alcohol/drug abuse and related emotional problems.	Weekly treatment consisted of 1 or 2 occupational therapy groups. Work-skills group: Long-term activities (e.g., leather, woodwork) and group discussion to improve participants' pre-work skills such as frustration tolerance, self-esteem, and direction following. Relationship-skills group: Participants worked together in activities (e.g., crafts, cooking) to develop relationship skills (e.g., leadership, socialization, expression of feelings). Outcome measure: Jamestown Occupational Therapy Assessment—rate general, interpersonal, and work behavior.	Participants who attended more occupational therapy sessions and participated in both groups were more likely to demonstrate change in behavioral area, particularly in relationship skills.	Rater bias might influence results. Nonstandardized measure Lack of control group Impact of other treatments in residential program not accounted for in analysis Outpatient group was offered only weekly visits.
http://dx.doi.org/10.1300/J004v07n02_06					
Gold et al. (2006)	To examine the effects of the inclusion of music therapy into standard care for children with autism spectrum disorders.	Level I—Systematic review. Three studies were reviewed; a total of 24 participants between the ages of 2 and 9 with a diagnosis of autism were included in the studies.	Intervention: Music therapy was the intervention in each study and included singing, listening to music, or playing an instrument. Outcome Measures: Observations of the following skills: • Nonverbal communication skills • Verbal communication skills • Frequency of problem behavior.	Medium effect size for improvements in nonverbal communication skills, and small to medium effect size for improvements in verbal communication skills. Improvements in music therapy were greater than effects of placebo therapy. Greater reductions in problematic behavior as a result of music therapy (small effect size) than reductions achieved as a result of placebo therapy.	No follow-up studies to determine long-term effects of treatment Two studies were not randomized. Blindness not reported in two studies Medications not monitored Short duration of studies
http://dx.doi.org/10.1002/14651858.CD004381.pub2					

Author/Year	Study Objectives	Level/Design/Participants	Intervention and Outcome Measures	Results	Study Limitations
Grizenko et al. (1993a) http://dx.doi.org/10.1097/00004583-199301000-00019	To examine differences in effect between day treatment and outpatient programs for children with disruptive behavior problems.	Level II—Cohort using repeated measures. 15 in day treatment—lived at home or in foster care; 15 in outpatient had received prior psychiatric services. Mean age 9 years (range 6–12 years) with severe behavior problem.	Day treatment provided multimodal therapy—special education, individual play therapy, systemic family therapy, and social-skills training. Outpatient treatment of weekly systemic therapy; several also were seen for individual play psychotherapy. Outcome Measures: • Revised Child Behaviour Profile • Children's Global Assessment Scale • Hare Self-Esteem Scale • Self-perception, peer relation, and family functioning—measured by Family Assessment Measure.	Day treatment was more effective for reducing problem behaviors perceived by parents and for improving child's secondary problems, such as difficulties with social skills and perceptions of themselves and their families.	Lack of random assignment No long-term follow-up included One-third of outpatient group had not completed therapy at 4-month outcome assessment period.
Grizenko et al. (1993b)	To evaluate efficacy of multimodal day treatment in addressing disruptive behavior in children.	Level II—Cohort using repeated measures. 15 in day treatment, 15 in wait-list control. Mean age 9 years (range 5–12 years). Diagnosis of ADHD, ODD, conduct disorder, or adjustment disorder with disturbances of conduct.	Day treatment intervention included special education, psychotherapy, individual play therapy, pet therapy, art therapy, occupational therapy, and family therapy. Outcome Measures: • Revised Child Behavior Profile • Self-perception and peer relationship (Hare Self-Esteem Scale, Hopelessness Scale, Index of Peer Relations) • Family Assessment Measure.	Attendance in day program led to significant reduction in child's expression of maladaptive behavior and increase in self-perception compared to children in control group. Significant difference was found in reintegration rate between 2 groups at the end of study period. No difference was found for peer relation, family functioning, and academics.	Lack of random assignment Small sample size Use of multimodal program may make it difficult to evaluate impact of an activity-based intervention.
Ikiugu & Ciaravino (2006)	To provide a preliminary test of the effectiveness of Instrumentalism in Occupational Therapy as a conceptual guide to intervention to help facilitate transition of adolescents with emotional and behavioral difficulties into adulthood.	Level III—Mixed-design pretest–posttest experimental study with naturalistic and phenomenological design. $N = 15$ (6 M, 9 F; 13–19 years old with learning disorder, attention deficit hyperactivity disorder, or serious conduct disorder)	Intervention methods, provided by occupational therapists, included collage making, goal setting, reading and listening activities, creating a poster, and a pizza-making activity. Outcome Measures: • Daily Activity Inventory • Occupational Performance Measure • Occupational Activity Classification; Allen Cognitive Levels Scale • Canadian Occupational Performance Measure (COPM) • Clarity of Desired Adult Life Assessment and Intervention Instrument for Instrumentalism in Occupational Therapy.	Significant increase in participation in occupations classified as neutral/decrease in frequency of participation in peer-related occupations, such as talking over the phone. Increased articulation of the value of friends and family. Correlation was found between increased COPM scores and increased frequency of neutral occupation participation.	Small sample size No control group—concurrent counseling sessions at the time of intervention Evaluators were not blinded to the treatment status.

(Continued)

Table C.3. Intensive Interventions

Author/Year	Study Objectives	Level/Design/Participants	Intervention and Outcome Measures	Results	Study Limitations
Ison (2001) http://dx.doi.org/10.2466/pr0.2001.88.3.903	To assess the efficacy of a social skills training program for children with conduct problems.	Level I—Randomized controlled trial. N = 315 children (164 = males with conduct problems, 151 = males without conduct problems) between the ages of 8 and 12 years old in Argentina. n = 171 treatment n = 174 control	Intervention: All treatment subgroups received social-skills training consisting of 14 teaching units (30 minutes/unit) two times per week. The control group did not receive social skills training. Outcome measures: • Self-Control Rating Scale • Child Behavior Report • Children's Behavioral Scenario.	Significant social improvements were found with the treatment groups in social skills by displaying a reduction in disruptive behaviors compared to the control group showing no change in behaviors in the Self-Control Rating Scale or Child Behavior Report.	Sample size limited in demographic representation and gender, reducing the generalizability of the conduct disorder population.
Kim et al. (2008) http://dx.doi.org/10.1007/s10803-008-0566-6	To evaluate the effectiveness of improvisational music therapy on joint attention behaviors of preschoolers with autism.	Level I—Randomized controlled trial. N = 10 children 3–5 years old with autism n = 5 music therapy sessions followed by play sessions n = 5 play sessions followed by music therapy	Interventions: Music therapy: Improvisational and used a variety of musical instruments Play: Used a variety of toys Outcome Measures: • Pervasive Developmental Disorder Behavior Inventory–C • Early Social Communication Scale.	Improvisational music therapy was more effective at facilitating joint attention behaviors and nonverbal social communication skills in children than play, along with significantly more and lengthier events of eye contact.	Small sample size High dropout rate
Koegel et al. (1987) http://dx.doi.org/10.1901/jaba.1987.20-243	To investigate whether engaging in child-preferred activities would be related to amount of social avoidance behavior exhibited by children with autism.	Level III—Before–after without control group. 10 participants diagnosed with mental retardation and autism with social avoidance behaviors. Ages 4–13 years.	Different adults in each session played with participants and changed toys about every minute. Outcome Measures: Observation of duration of child-preferred behavior and social avoidance behaviors, and social responsiveness.	Social avoidance behaviors decreased when children with autism were prompted to initiate appropriate child-preferred activities.	Reliability of independent variable (play with participants) not measured. Small sample size No control group

Kroeger et al. (2007)	To investigate the effectiveness of group-delivered social skills interventions (direct group instruction, free play, video modeling) for young children with autism.	Level II—Nonrandomized control study. 25 4- to 6-year-old children diagnosed with autism $n = 13$ direct instruction $n = 12$ free play	Interventions: Direct instruction—social skills, video modeling of social skills Control: Free play. Groups meet for 5 weeks, 3 times per week, for an hour each session. Outcome Measures: • Social Observation Code videotape data • Assessment of Basic Language and Learning Skills • Parent Satisfaction Rating Scale.	Both groups improved on their prosocial behaviors, behaviors of initiation, and maintain social interaction from pre- to posttest. The direct-instruction group showed significant gains in social skills when compared to the play activities group. Both groups increased their learning readiness. No significant difference was found between the satisfaction of parents from either group.	Small sample size No blinding of researchers No randomization
http://dx.doi.org/10.1007/s10803-006-0207-x					
Laugeson et al. (2009)	To examine the effect of the Program for the Education and Enrichment of Relational Skills (PEERS) on improving peer interactions, such as the quality of friendships and social skills on teens age 13–17 diagnosed with high-functioning autism spectrum disorder (HFASD).	Level 1—Randomized controlled trial. $N = 36$ 13- to 17-year-olds with HFASD $n = 17$ PEERS $n = 16$ delayed treatment control (3 dropouts)	Intervention included sessions providing education to parents and teens on making and keeping friends followed by modeling using role play. Control: Delayed treatment. Outcome Measures: • Vineland Adaptive Behavior Scales • Social Skills Rating Scale • Quality of Play Questionnaire Test of Adolescent Social Skills Knowledge • Friendship Quality Scale	The treatment group demonstrated a significant increase in hosted get-togethers and significant improvement of parent-reported social skills, along with significantly better quality of friendships. The delayed-treatment group demonstrated significantly decreased friendship quality.	Short treatment period of only 12 weeks Teacher reports were received from only 13 out of 33 subjects. Parent-reported outcomes may have been biased due to not being blinded to intervention.
http://dx.doi.org/10.1007/s10803-008-0664-5					
Lee et al. (2007)	To evaluate the effectiveness of self-management for students with autism.	Level 1—Meta-analysis of single-subject design studies. Searched PsycINFO, ERIC and Wilson OmniFile for studies published prior to 2004. Total of 11 articles with 34 participants. Excluded teenagers and preschoolers.	The studies of self-management included prompting, social-skills training, discriminative training, and self-monitoring Outcome Measure: Appropriate behaviors such as social communication and interaction, schedule following, learning daily living skills.	Although there were differences for self-management techniques (in particular studies that used coparticipants), there were no statistically significant differences.	Small number of participants included in review
http://dx.doi.org/10.1177/10883576070220010101					

(Continued)

Table C.3. Intensive Interventions

Author/Year	Study Objectives	Level/Design/Participants	Intervention and Outcome Measures	Results	Study Limitations
LeGoff (2004)	To determine the effects of LEGO social skills group on social competence.	Level II—Nonrandomized trial; subjects served as own controls. Children with autistic disorder, Asperger syndrome, or pervasive developmental disorder not otherwise specified; $N = 47$ (34 M, 13 F). Mean age = 10.6 years and 10.10 years for the two groups.	Intervention: LEGO therapy included the following elements: children played with LEGOs and followed simple social rules, points were awarded for appropriate social behaviors, siblings attended as helpers, group members made joint decisions, and families developed a support network. Outcome Measures: • Count of number of self-initiated social contact • Duration of social interactions • Social Interaction subscale of the Gilliam Autism Rating Scale (GAS).	Significant differences were found between treatment and control phases for all three dependent variables. All (social initiation, duration of social interactions, and social interaction per the GAS) showed significant improvement following the LEGO therapy. There was a 175% increase in duration of social interaction with peers in free play.	Nonrandomized sample Limited description of LEGO therapy Lack of theoretical basis for study, which limits generalizability
http://dx.doi.org/10.1007/s10803-004-2550-0					
LeGoff & Sherman (2006)	To compare social competence and autistic behaviors in children who received LEGO therapy and those who received comparable social-skills interventions and to examine variables that predict outcome.	Level II—Retroactive pre-post control group design using a matched sample of two groups of nonrandomized children. Subjects: $N = 117$, 60 in the LEGO group (49 M), 57 in the control group (47 M). The children were diagnosed with autistic disorder ($n = 50$), Asperger syndrome ($n = 55$), or pervasive developmental disorder not otherwise specified ($n = 12$).	Intervention: In the LEGO intervention, children participated in a LEGO club, where they learn to collaborate to build LEGO structures. The control group received the same amount and types of individual and group therapy as the children in the LEGO therapy. Outcome Measures: • Vineland Adaptive Behavior social domain • Gilliam Autism Rating Scale (GARS), Social Interaction scale • Secondary analysis used the Wechsler IQ, Vineland Adaptive Behavior composite, and Wechsler verbal IQ.	A significant interaction between time (pre- and post-test) and group (control and LEGO) revealed that the LEGO group improved more on the Vineland Social domain and scored lower (improved) on the GARS Social Interaction scale. Secondary analyses indicated that the child's function level at the beginning predicted social adaptive behaviors. Language function also predicted social competency outcomes. Language predicted outcomes more for the Asperger group than for the autistic disorder group.	The intervention was not well described. This retrospective study used data that had been collected in the past (documents/records). The samples were nonrandomized. The evaluator (first author) was not blind to group assignment.
http://dx.doi.org/10.1177/1362361306064403					

Lopata et al. (2008)	To replicate the findings of a manualized social treatment program for children with high-functioning autism spectrum disorder (HFASD)	Level 1—Randomized controlled trial. $N = 54$ children (50 M, 4 F) between the ages of 6–13 with a diagnosis of HFASD $n = 25$ Response Cost (RC) $n = 29$ Noncategorical (NC)	Intervention: Both groups participated in face emotion recognition, social-skills groups, and therapeutic activity to practice skill. RC group received performance feedback by earning or losing points. The NC group received feedback not based on predetermined behavioral categories. Outcome Measures: • Behavior Assessment System for Children (BASC) • BASC Parent Rating Scales • BASC Teacher Rating Scales.	Significant improvements were found for the overall program for social skills and problem behaviors; however, there were no findings to support the superiority of one feedback format over the other. There was no difference for face emotion recognition.	Sample size was limited in terms of size and demographic representation, thus restricting generalizability. Lack of a no-treatment control group Lack of a "gold standard" autism diagnostic instrument during sample selection

http://dx.doi.org/10.1007/s10803-007-0460-7

Machalicek et al. (2007)	To examine effectiveness of procedures used to reduce challenging behaviors of children with autism spectrum disorder (ASD) in school settings	Level 1—Meta-analysis. $N = 1$–5 3- to 17-year-olds with ASD Single-subject design studies published between 1995–2005.	Ten studies manipulated antecedent conditions using social stories, video modeling, exercise, and cue card strategies. Five studies changed instructional content by using prompting strategies, embedded instruction, therapy balls as seats, rhythmic entrainment, and choice of reinforcements. Eight studies used differential reinforcement of other behaviors; five of these studies used functional communication training. Three studies used self-management strategies. Outcome Measure: Assessment of frequency of challenging behaviors.	85% of the studies reported decreases in challenging behaviors secondary to the interventions they used. Antecedent manipulations, changes in instructional content, differential reinforcement, and self-management strategies all appeared to be effective interventions. Although some studies showed positive results for decreased behaviors, the participants in these studies still demonstrated undesirable behaviors.	Findings of some of the individual studies in this group provided results that are unclear as to whether the interventions are effective, and one showed that specific interventions cannot be interpreted as effective due to conditions during the study. Some of the studies with positive results did not give unequivocal data. The authors reported that interpretations of the results of the studies included in this meta-analysis were questionable. All studies were single-subject design.

http://dx.doi.org/10.1080/13668250701689280

(Continued)

Table C.3. Intensive Interventions

Author/Year	Study Objectives	Level/Design/Participants	Intervention and Outcome Measures	Results	Study Limitations
Mackay et al. (2007)	To enhance social interaction and understanding in high-functioning children and adolescents with autism spectrum disorder (ASD) through a group intervention.	Level III—One-group, nonrandomized, pre- and posttest. N = 46 children/adolescents with ASD between the ages of 6–12 (38 Male, 6 Female).	Intervention: Groups included social and emotional perspective-taking, conversation skills, and friendship skills. Groups included games and role play. 1½ hour weekly sessions over 12–16 weeks. Outcome Measures: • The Spence Social Skills Questionnaire • Social Competence Questionnaires • Individual parent rating scale.	Enhanced levels of functioning for social skills and social competence were reported by both parents and subjects.	Lack of control group Cannot generalize results to any specific subgroup within ASD Different groups were led by different staff members.
http://dx.doi.org/10.1080/13668250701689280					
Owens et al. (2008)	To compare the effectiveness of two social skills programs: LEGO therapy and Social Use of Language Programme (SULP).	Level 1—Randomized controlled trial. N = 31 children (30 Male, 1 Female) between the ages of 6 and 11 years with a diagnosis of high-functioning autism, autism spectrum disorder, autism, or Asperger syndrome. n = 16 LEGO n = 15 SULP n = 16 no intervention (matched on age, IQ and severity)	Intervention: LEGO: Collaborating in LEGO play. SULP: Teaching approach based around stories, group activities, and games. Groups were held for 1 hr per week for 18 weeks. A nonintervention control group was recruited at a later date. Outcome Measures: • Vineland Adaptive Behavior Scale • Gilliam Autism Rating Scale Social Interaction subscale.	A reduction in autism-specific social difficulties was seen following LEGO therapy, in contrast to no changes in the SULP or control groups. Significant results were found for both LEGO therapy and SULP in reducing maladaptive behavior.	No random assignment in control group Potential bias: Outcome measures were completed by parents, who were aware of what intervention their child was receiving. The same researcher also ran both interventions. No treatment fidelity measures were taken. Reduced generalizability due to small sample size and predominantly male subjects
http://dx.doi.org/10.1007/s10803-008-0590-6					

Study	Purpose / Level / Participants	Intervention / Outcome Measures	Results	Limitations
Ozonoff & Miller (1995) http://dx.doi.org/10.1007/BF02179376	To examine effectiveness of social-skills training program for normal-IQ adolescents with autism. Level II—Nonrandomized controlled trial. 5 participants; all participants with autism were male. Mean ages 13.8 years in treatment group ($n = 1$) and 13.6 years in control group ($n = 4$).	Social-skills training program (experimental group) included daily topic discussions, role-play for modeling skills, coaching from trainers, videotaped role-plays, and games. Outcome Measure: Social cognition and social skill by Theory of Mind Tasks and Social Skills Rating System.	Social-skills training program providing systematic instruction in theory of mind principles (ability to attribute mental states to others) was able to improve performance on several false-belief tasks. However, it failed to improve social competence for participants on parent and teacher ratings.	Small sample size Lack of random assignment Treatment program period might be too short to facilitate participants' social skills.
Sachs & Miller (2001)	To examine impact of wilderness experience on social interactions and expectations of adolescents with behavior disorders. Level I—Randomized controlled trial. 8 in experimental group, 8 in control group. Ages 13–17 years (mean age 16 years). Diagnosis of behavior disorder.	Intervention: Wilderness camping trip including hiking, trail making, problem solving, trust and relaxation activities. Control activities: Relaxation training, increased free time, and movies. Outcome Measures: • Direct observation • Behavior Problem Checklist • Modified Jessup Expectancy Questionnaire.	Wilderness camping experience had short-term effects on cooperation of treatment group. Although no difference existed at follow-up on outcome measures, experimental group continued to cooperate more on average than control group.	Small sample size Attrition of 1 experimental and 2 control participants strongly affected results given small sample size.
Schleien et al. (1990)	To explore effects of using four social levels of play on appropriate play behavior of children with autism in integrated leisure education/ physical education program. Level III—Before–after. 17 participants with autism (ages 5–12 years) with social withdrawal and severe communication disorder; 21 nondisabled students served as peer group.	16 recreational activities represented 4 levels of structured play (isolate, dyadic, group, and team play). Positive reinforcement was provided to participants with autism for facilitating appropriate play behaviors. Outcome Measure: Two observers independently recorded appropriate play behavior during each play session.	Structured integrated activities involving higher levels of social play elicited significantly higher frequency of appropriate play behavior in school-age students with autism.	Small sample size Lack of control group Treatment effect due to nature of play activities or presence of nondisabled students as peers was unknown.

(Continued)

Table C.3. Intensive Interventions

Author/Year	Study Objectives	Level/Design/Participants	Intervention and Outcome Measures	Results	Study Limitations
Schleien et al. (1995) http://dx.doi.org/10.1007/BF02179375	To evaluate effect of art activities on cooperation and social interaction for children with and without autism.	Level III—Before–after (with multiple baseline). 15 children with autism with or without moderate/severe mental retardation, Rett's syndrome. Older group—7 (mean age 9 years), younger group—8 (mean age 6 years). 53 nondisabled children also participated in study as special friends of autistic child.	Following baseline art sessions, nondisabled peers participated in session that introduced ways to interact with children with autism. Each autistic participant was matched with 3 or 4 nondisabled peers and participated in 6 monthly art activities. Outcome Measure: Observers recorded appropriate/ inappropriate behavior and social interaction of children with autism.	Interactions initiated by students with autism toward nondisabled peers did not change significantly before and after intervention. Nondisabled participants demonstrated greater social interaction toward peers with autism during art activities than before intervention.	Lack of control group Rate of positive interactions per minute varied greatly from session to session, perhaps because of nature of art activities developed in program. Lack of evaluation of generalization to school setting Lack of clear understanding of amount and type of art program needed to facilitate interactions for participants
Stermac & Josefowitz (1985) http://dx.doi.org/10.1007/s10803-006-0343-3	To evaluate effects of playing therapeutic board game on social skills of severely behaviorally disordered adolescents.	Level III—Before–after. 7 adolescents (ages 13–17 years) in a day treatment program for adolescents with mental disorder who were identified by staff as having severe cognitive and social deficits that precluded participation in traditional group psychotherapy.	Social Skills Board Game devised by day treatment staff that required drawing cards on social dilemmas, such as asking someone for directions. Situations were role-played with feedback and ideas given by staff and peers. Outcome Measures: • Participants were videotaped role playing a standard set of 6 scenarios before and after intervention. • Rating of behavior was done by trained researchers.	Social skills improved, and bizarre behavior decreased.	Small sample size Measures used were not standardized. Use of multimodal program may make it difficult to evaluate impact of 1 activity-based intervention. Lack of control group
Tse et al. (2007)	To determine the effectiveness of a social skills training program on social competence for adolescents with Asperger syndrome and high-functioning autism (AS/HFA)	Level III—Pretest–posttest design. N = 46 adolescents age 13–18 with AS/HFA in Montreal, Canada.	Intervention: The group social-skills curriculum consisted of psychoeducational and experiential methods of teaching social skills, with emphasis on learning through role play. Outcome Measures: • The Social Responsiveness Scale • Aberrant Behavior Checklist • Nisonger Child Behavior Rating Scale • Feedback survey.	Significant pre- to posttreatment gains were found on measures of both social competence and problem behaviors associated with AS/HFA. Effect sizes ranged from 0.34 to 0.72. Adolescents reported more perceived skill improvements than did parents. Parent-reported improvement suggests that social skills learned in group sessions generalize to settings outside the treatment group.	Lack of a control group Group program not manualized Use of parent-report measure for quantitative measurement

Citation	Purpose	Study design/level of evidence	Intervention and outcome measures	Results	Study limitations
Wood et al. (2009) http://dx.doi.org/10.1007/s10803-009-0791-7	To evaluate the effectiveness of cognitive–behavioral therapy (CBT) on parent-reported autism symptoms.	Level 1—Randomized controlled trial. N = 19 children with high-functioning autism spectrum disorders and an anxiety disorder n = 9 CBT n = 10 wait-list control	Intervention: Building Confidence, a CBT program, emphasized *in vivo* exposure supported by parent training and school consultation. Wait-list control group Outcome Measures: • Social Responsiveness Scale • Anxiety Disorders Interview Scale.	Participants in the CBT group outperformed the wait-list group at posttreatment/postwait-list on total parent-reported autism symptoms. Treatment gains were maintained at 3-month follow-up.	Small sample size Parent reports of symptomatology

Note. ADD = attention deficit disorder; ADHD = attention deficit hyperactivity disorder; ODD = oppositional defiant disorder

Appendix D. Supplementary Information Related to Children's Mental Health

The following supplemental information focuses on topics relevant to occupational therapy's role in mental health promotion, prevention, and intervention with children and youth. The first three sections provide information relevant to occupational therapy intervention, including mental health literacy, sensory processing, and participation in structured leisure occupations. The final three sections focus on a selection of situational factors associated with mental health challenges: bullying and friendship issues, obesity, and risky teen behavior. Occupational therapy practitioners need to consider how to develop targeted services for these and other at-risk groups in order to prevent mental health challenges and promote positive mental health.

Mental Health Literacy

Mental health literacy focuses on providing all children and youth with a working knowledge of mental health as an integral part of overall health (Barry & Jenkins, 2007). The term *mental health literacy* was introduced in Australia by Anthony Jorm and represents a relatively new area of study (Jorm et al., 1997). It is a concept derived from the term *health literacy:* the functional capacity to understand and use information for the purpose of personal health promotion. *Mental health literacy* refers to the knowledge and beliefs about mental health and mental disorders, which assists in knowing how to foster mental health as well as to

recognize, manage, and seek treatment for mental illness (Griffiths, Christensen, & Jorm, 2009).

As a Tier 1 service, a school-based occupational therapy practitioner might collaborate with health educators, school nurses, or guidance counselors in coteaching a unit on the mental health continuum, including mental illness, languishing, moderate mental health, and flourishing (Keyes, 2007). Programs that help children learn and talk about mental health, mental illness, and interventions may help reduce the negative stigma associated with mental illness by helping bring the topic into everyday conversations and framing mental health as a positive state of functioning. Developing and implementing whole-school strategies to teach children and youth about positive mental health might be organized for the Substance Abuse and Mental Health Services Administration's National Children's Mental Health Awareness Day, which occurs annually in May. The use of posters, bookmarks, coloring sheets, and even handwriting sheets that communicate strategies for taking care of one's mental health can be embedded in everyday practice to promote mental health literacy.

Sensory Processing

With a strong knowledge base in sensory processing, an occupational therapist is often one of the only members of interdisciplinary teams to recognize the implications of sensory processing disorders on social, emotional, and physical function. "Occupational therapy practitioners recognize that well-regulated sensory systems can contribute to important outcomes in social–emotional, physical, communication, self-care, cognitive, and adaptive skill development" (AOTA, 2008, p.1). Occupational therapists' specific knowledge and skill in this area can be applied at universal, targeted, and intensive levels to promote successful participation in school, home, and community settings for children with and without disabilities. A guiding belief is that all children and adults are sensory beings responding to everyday sensation in individual ways, resulting in unique sensory preferences that are reflected in what they do and how they interact with others.

Although most people demonstrate mild or moderate responses to sensory input (e.g., mild irritation in a crowded mall), allowing for successful participation throughout the day, those with various disabilities (e.g., autism) or mental illness (e.g., psychosis) may respond to sensory input in more intense ways, resulting in performance challenges (Dunn, 2007). Intense responses to sensory input, for example, can negatively influence a person's emotions (e.g., causing irritability or tantrums) and social interaction (e.g., causing withdrawal or aggression). Occupational therapy practitioners can play an important role in helping children, families, and professionals develop a working knowledge of sensory processing in order to understand children's behaviors and modify everyday interactions and environments to foster success and well-being (Dunn, 2007).

A wealth of information in the form of journal articles, books, workshops, and Internet resources is available to assist occupational therapists in the evaluation and intervention of sensory processing disorders, especially at the intensive and targeted levels. The authors also acknowledge that the evidence presented in this document is presented within the context of children's mental health. Individuals seeking detailed evidence on sensory

processing can refer to AOTA's Practice Guideline that focuses on this topic: *Occupational Therapy Practice Guidelines for Children and Adolescents With Challenges in Sensory Processing and Sensory Integration* (Watling, Koenig, Davies, & Schaaf, 2011) provides a comprehensive perspective on the current evidence on sensory processing and sensory integration.

At the universal level, growing attention to the importance of education (Dunn, 2007) and environmental modifications (Champagne, 2008; Vogel, 2008) is occurring in order to enhance an understanding of and respect for sensory differences as well as to create environments that support a sense of comfort and emotional well-being. Table D.1 provides examples of sensory processing promotion, prevention, and intervention strategies and resources. Applying knowledge at each level of service requires the use of a broad range of strategies, including direct (individual or group interventions) and indirect (in-service education, consultation with teachers and families, environmental modifications).

Structured Leisure Participation

An important aspect of occupation-based practice when working with children and youth is attention to the development of structured leisure participation during out-of-school time. Youth participation in structured leisure, such as sports teams, clubs, and lessons, is relatively common, with approximately 6 in 10 youth participating in organized out-of-school activities at any given time (Mahoney et al., 2005, 2008). It is important for occupational therapy practitioners to be aware of the multiple benefits of such participation and help children develop health leisure interests.

Structured leisure participation enhances personal development in several ways (Hansen et al., 2003). First, participation provides opportunities to facilitate *identity work*. Exposure to and participation in a variety of leisure activities allows

Table D.1. Application of Sensory Processing Within a Public Health Model

Tier	Emphasis	Examples of Resources
Tier 3: Intensive, individualized • Children and youth with identified sensory processing challenges	• Evaluate individuals: Identify patterns of sensory processing (overresponsive, underresponsive) and impact on participation. • Use interventions on the basis of individualized need and setting: In schools, interventions are generally embedded within school environment (classroom, cafeteria). Example: Develop a sensory diet for the child. • Educate to enhance understanding about the meaning of behavior from a sensory perspective.	Assessments (examples, not an inclusive list): • Sensory Processing Measure (Miller-Kuhanek, Henry, Glennon, Parham, & Ecker, 2008) • Sensory Profile (Dunn, 1999) Sensory and environmental modifications applied in mental health: • Sensory Modulation Program; restraint reduction (Tina Champagne); www.ot-innovations.com • Sensory Connection Program (Karen M. Moore); www.sensoryconnectionprogram.com
Tier 2: Selective • Small group • Targeted	• Screen at-risk children and youth for possible sensory processing challenges (e.g., autism spectrum disorder, anxiety disorders, those experiencing prodromal symptoms). • Modify environments (e.g., classroom, cafeteria, playground, home) to meet a range of sensory needs.	Evaluation: Observation in natural context; interviews of parents and teachers Intervention resources: • *The Alert Program: How Does Your Engine Run?* (Williams & Shellenberger, 1996) • *The Tool Chest: For Teachers, Parents and Students* (Henry, 2001)
Tier 1: Universal • Whole school • Community	• Educate children, youth, families, and professionals about sensory processing, impact on behavior, and accommodations. • Evaluate environments for design qualities to promote social participation and learning.	• In-services or presentations to children and youth, teachers and other school staff, and parent groups • Serve on committees addressing school and community environmental design to address sensory variables in cafeteria, play areas, hallways, and classrooms

Note. From "Major Approaches Useful in Addressing the Mental Health Needs of Children and Youth" by S. Bazyk, in *Mental Health Promotion, Prevention, and Intervention With Children and Youth: A Guiding Framework for Occupational Therapy* (p. 59), by S. Bazyk (Ed.) 2011b, Bethesda, MD, the American Occupational Therapy Association. Copyright © 2011. Reprinted with permission.

a young person to explore, express, and refine his or her identity and passion (Kleiber, 1999). During such participation, youth assess their talents, interests, values, and place in the social structure. Second, organized activities have been viewed as providing a context for the development of *initiative* (Larson, 2000). According to Larson (2000), initiative reflects the self-motivation needed to devote effort over time to achieve a challenging goal—a core quality individuals need in order to deal with the complexities of adult life and future work. Three elements of initiative include (a) *intrinsic motivation* (wanting to do the activity), (b) *concerted engagement,* and (c) *commitment over time.* The third domain of personal development

includes cognitive, physical, and emotional skills (Hansen et al., 2003). Participation in organized activities is associated with higher academic achievement (Passmore, 1998); the development of positive habits contributing to physical health, especially with sports (Mahoney et al., 2005); skill development (e.g., athletic, artistic, homemaking); and beginning work skills (Dworkin, 2003; Mahoney & Stattin, 2000). Several emotional competencies have been associated with participation in structured leisure, including managing feelings, controlling impulses, and increasing self-esteem (Mahoney et al., 2005). In terms of emotional wellbeing, Csikszentmihalyi (1993) found that when people learn to enjoy complex occupations that provide challenges corresponding to their skills, they are more likely to develop innate abilities, experience a positive self-esteem, and be happier overall.

Interpersonal development also focuses on the development of social connections. Structured leisure activities involve higher social complexity requiring peer cooperation and the guidance of adult role models. First, participation in organized activities provides an important context for the development of new peer friendships—often with youth who attend different schools and from varying ethnicities and social classes (Dworkin et al., 2003). Second, youth activities provide opportunities to develop a variety of social skills, including working effectively with others, giving and receiving feedback, and acquiring appropriate values about rules and conduct across settings (Hansen et al., 2003; Mahoney et al., 2005). A third attribute of interpersonal development is the growth of close connections to adults with social capital, such as coaches, artists, dancers, musicians, and other valued community members. These relationships can become long-term sources of emotional and social capital (e.g., access to information about future jobs or colleges; McLaughlin, 2000).

To "derive the greatest benefits from organized activities, a youth must participate" (Mahoney et al., 2005, p. 13). Both exposure to a range of potential leisure occupations and the availability of resources to support engagement are critical factors influencing the likelihood that children and adolescents will develop and maintain healthy leisure interests. "Availability and affordability of activities are the most basic factors affecting participation" (Mahoney et al., 2005, p. 14). Resources such as parks, organized sports and other community programs, and competent adults to oversee the activities are essential. The provision of transportation and financial support also are crucial factors influencing participation.

Given the developmental and mental health benefits of participation in structured leisure, there are many ways in which occupational therapy services can be provided to promote meaningful leisure participation for all children. First and foremost, occupational therapists can advocate for participation in structured leisure for all children by educating young people, families, teachers, and community leaders about the benefits of leisure participation. Special efforts to promote participation might be necessary for children at risk of limited participation because of restricted access and availability (e.g., low-income urban youth, children with disabilities). Occupational therapy practitioners might assume the role of "leisure coach" with youth deprived of leisure participation opportunities or develop group programs to promote participation in structured leisure pursuits.

Bullying and Friendship Issues

Bullying is considered one of the most common forms of violence in schools, and therefore most schools adopt programs to reduce bullying and create physically and emotionally safe contexts for learning (Collaborative for Academic, Social, and Emotional Learning [CASEL], 2009, Espelage & Swearer, 2003; Nansel et al., 2001). In addition, 46 states (as of June 2011) have passed anti-bullying laws, including clear prohibitions on bullying and legislative findings of its negative effects on school environments (see http://bullypolice.org).

Although many definitions have been proposed, the Center for the Study and Prevention of School Violence (2008) described *bullying* as an act of intentional aggression carried out repeatedly over time and occurring within a relationship characterized by an imbalance of power. Three types of bullying have been identified: (a) *direct* (e.g., pushing, shoving), (b) *indirect* (e.g., spreading negative rumors), and (c) *cyberbullying* (e.g., negative remarks about a person posted on an Internet site). Boys tend to be involved in more direct acts of bullying, whereas girls are more likely to engage in indirect forms (Jenson & Dieterich, 2007). Because indirect and cyberbullying are less visible to external parties, it is often difficult for adults to detect and address such behavior (Nansel et al., 2001).

In 2007, approximately 32% of students (ages 12–18) reported being bullied within the past year, with 63% of these bullied one to two times over the year, 21% bullied one to two times per month, 10% bullied one to two times per week, and 7% bullied almost daily (CASEL, 2009). Bullying tends to peak between ages 11 and 13 years and continues to decline throughout the high school grades (CASEL, 2009; Jenson & Dieterich, 2007).

Several mental health risks are associated with victims, bullies, and bystanders. Victims of bullying report symptoms of emotional distress, including low self-esteem, loneliness, depression, anxiety, and poor academic performance (Jenson & Dieterich, 2007). Children who bully often display a range of negative outcomes, including poor school adjustment, conduct problems, depression, and peer rejection. In addition, bystanders who witness bullying can experience feelings of fear, anger, guilt, and sadness (Batsche & Porter, 2006). Bystanders also may play a role in acting in ways to maintain bullying behavior by either responding positively (e.g., laughing, joining in) or by passively watching rather than intervening to help the victim. Although most discussions of bullying generally label individuals as bully or victim, some researchers suggest that bullying should be viewed along a continuum and as a group phenomenon that occurs in a social context (CASEL, 2009). For example, most students experience moments of both throughout their development—partaking in some form of bullying and being teased or harassed by peers at some point (Espelage & Swearer, 2003).

Schoolwide Bully Prevention Programs

Because bullying can affect the entire student body and school climate, existing research supports universal school-based programs as opposed to involving only victims and bullies. According to several researchers in the area (Swearer, Espelage, Love, & Kingsbury, 2008; Ttofi & Farrington, 2009; Vreeman & Carroll, 2007), effective whole-school approaches consist of a variety of strategies, such as teacher training, schoolwide rules, classroom curricula and management strategies, parent education, improved playground supervision, and peer involvement to combat bullying.

Embedding bully prevention within schoolwide social and emotional learning (SEL) and positive behavioral support (PBS) has been proposed (CASEL, 2009; OSEP Technical Assistance Center on Positive Behavioral Interventions and Supports, n.d). Bully prevention in PBS emphasizes remediation of problem behavior and *prevention* of further bullying. Two bully prevention program manuals, one for elementary and the other for middle school, are available on the OSEP Technical Assistance Center on Positive Behavioral Interventions and Supports Web site (see Box D.1).

Bully prevention within an SEL framework emphasizes the promotion of a positive school climate (warmth, respect) and positive student interactions (increasing SEL competencies). Students who have greater SEL competency are less likely to be aggressors, targets of bullying, or passive bystanders. In addition, schools that create positive schoolwide environments are not conducive to bullying, making such behaviors less likely to occur or continue. A document describing an SEL and bullying prevention framework is available on the CASEL Web site (www.casel.org). It appears that a combination of PBS and SEL approaches would provide a comprehensive way to ensure the prevention of bullying and the promotion of skills emphasizing positive interaction.

Occupational therapy practitioners need to become aware of state and district policies and approaches for addressing bullying and actively support such efforts by embedding school- and classroom-wide strategies into occupational therapy intervention when possible. Special attention to the

Bully Prevention in Positive Behavioral Interventions and Supports (BP–PBIS) was designed to augment schoolwide PBIS by teaching all students behaviors that will reduce the probability of bullying. The program emphasizes prevention and remediation of the problem. BP–PBIS gives students the tools necessary to remove the social rewards maintaining inappropriate behavior, thereby decreasing the likelihood of problem behavior occurring in the future. The manuals provide clear methods and user-friendly worksheets for teaching this program to students and staff.

Students are taught a three-step response to problem behavior to prevent the reinforcement of bullying and to extinguish it. Separate sections apply the three steps to the problems of gossip, inappropriate remarks, and cyberbullying:

1. *Stop:* Teach students the schoolwide "stop signal" (verbal and physical action) for problem behavior, and practice when and how to use it appropriately.
2. *Walk:* Teach students to walk away when the problem behavior continues after the stop signal. Walking away removes the reinforcement for problem behavior.
3. *Talk:* Teach students to talk to an adult if the problem behavior continues after using stop and walk.

Staff (e.g., teachers, paraprofessionals, administrators) are taught a clear and simple method of responding to reports of problem behavior and delivering consequences.

See the *Bully Prevention Manuals* (available for free online at www.pbis.org) for a complete description of the program.

Source. Stiller, Ross, and Horner (n.d.-a, n.d.-b).

Note. From "Enduring Challenges and Situational Stessors During the School Years: Risk Reduction and Competence Enhancement" (p. 125), by S. Bazyk in *Mental Health Promotion, Prevention, and Intervention With Children and Youth: A Guiding Framework for Occupational Therapy*, (p. 125), by S. Bazyk (Ed.) 2011a, Bethesda, MD: AOTA Press. Copyright © 2011 by the American Occupational Therapy Association. Reprinted with permission.

development of skills important for developing and sustaining friendships easily can be embedded into occupational therapy services.

Children with disabilities are often targets of bullying because of their differences (Heinrich, 2003). Those diagnosed with special needs, such as ADHD, oppositional defiant disorder, bipolar disorder, obsessive–compulsive disorder, a nonverbal learning disability, Asperger syndrome, and/or a learning disorder may experience anxiety and depression and are typically more rejected by their peers. It is essential that adaptations and modifications be integrated into bullying prevention programs as necessary to successfully meet the requirements of children with special needs.

Promotion of Friendship Skills

Research suggests that having high-quality friendships, or at least one best friend, can help prevent children from being a victim of bullying (CASEL, 2009). In addition, friendships are also an important source of happiness (Demir, Zdemir, & Weitekamp, 2007). Friendship is a qualitative relationship that represents voluntary interdependence over time and involves varying degrees of companionship, affection, intimacy, and mutual assistance. Recent research suggests that close friendships contribute to happiness above and beyond the influence of one's personality (Demir & Weitekamp, 2007). In addition, the companionship and self-validation features of friendship were found to be the most important predictors of happiness.

Companionship refers to doing things with friends—sharing in activities perceived as enjoyable or exciting. *Self-validation*, the second feature of friendship associated with happiness, refers to perceiving the friend as being supportive of one's self-image by listening, agreeing, reassuring, and encouraging (e.g., gives compliments, points out strengths; Demir & Weitekamp, 2007). In addition to the relationship between friendships and happiness, children who have friends tend to be more sociable, self-confident, cooperative, and emotionally supportive than those without friends (Wentzel, Baker, & Russell, 2009).

Occupational therapy practitioners can play a pivotal role in helping all children and youth develop friendships both in and out of school. The first step is asking children about their friends and friendship issues. Informal interviews and observations of children and youth in natural settings is one way to gather information about friendship skills. Attwood (2002) identified social behaviors important for friendship development (e.g., knowing how to enter a group, giving compliments at appropriate times, demonstrating empathy). Occupational therapy intervention can help teach friendship skills during individual or group interaction. To foster the development of friends outside of school, it is important to help children identify their interests and join a group or club. The use of coaching strategies can assist children who are reluctant or who have limited social skills to successfully enter and participate in a group. Doing enjoyable activities with other children increases the opportunity to develop friends with those who have similar interests.

Obesity

Obesity is a major public health concern in the United States and other Western countries. Approximately 34.3% of U.S. adults 20 years and older are overweight, 33.8% are obese, and 5.7% are extremely obese (Centers for Disease Control and Prevention, 2010). Of significant concern is the growing rate of childhood obesity, with about 25% of children being overweight and 11% being obese (Dehghan, Akhtar-Danesh, & Merchant, 2005; Dwyer, Baur, Higgs, & Hardy, 2009).

Causes

Overall, the combined effect of overconsumption of calories and reduced physical activity is considered the biggest cause of childhood obesity (Dehghan et al., 2005). Societal influences, such as the overavailability of foods high in sugar and fat, increased size of food servings, increased time spent in television- and computer-related activities, and decreased physical activity, have contributed to the obesity epidemic (AOTA, 2013). The decrease in physical activity can be attributed, in part, to less time spent in physical education class and recess, decreased time spent in outside play, and increased use of automated transportation (Smallfield & Anderson, 2009).

Children at Greater Risk of Obesity

Children living in poverty and those with disabilities are at even greater risk for becoming overweight or obese at young ages, making this a social justice issue as well as a public health epidemic. Youth growing up in low-income urban environments in working-class African American and Latino communities have rates of obesity almost double those of White children (Cahill & Suarez-Balcazar, 2009). Such environments generally provide fewer opportunities for physical activity (e.g., fewer safe public play areas) and less access to nutritional foods (prevalence of fast food outlets and convenience stores vs. grocery stores).

The prevalence of overweight and obesity is higher among children with developmental disabilities (40%) than in the general population, leading to a greater number of obesity-related secondary conditions (e.g., fatigue, pain, deconditioning, social isolation, difficulty performing activities of daily living; De, Small, & Baur, 2008; Rimmer, Rowland, & Yamaki, 2007). Children with developmental disabilities often have one or more predisposing factors for obesity, including the coexistence of certain genetic syndromes known to be associated with obesity (Prader–Willi syndrome), reduced levels of physical activity, and the use of medications that can cause weight gain (De et al., 2008). Factors within the physical and social environments, such as a lack of access to recreation facilities and limited knowledge among staff on how to adapt programs for youth with disabilities, also may contribute to a lack of physical activity (Rimmer et al., 2007). Finally, research has shown that, by age 3 years, children with developmental delay are significantly more likely to be obese than their typically developing peers (Emerson, 2009). Such findings make a case for the investment in interventions during the early years of life to prevent the emergence of obesity among children with developmental delay. It is important for occupational therapy practitioners to be aware of conditions that put children at greater risk of obesity and embed into their interventions strategies to prevent obesity and promote health.

Consequences

Obesity in childhood is known to have a significant impact on physical and emotional health as well as social interaction (Smallfield & Anderson, 2009). Physically, obesity is linked to an increased risk for diabetes, heart disease, high cholesterol, high blood pressure, sleep apnea, and orthopedic problems. Emotionally, children who are obese may experience negative effects associated with weight bias. *Weight bias* refers to weight-related attitudes and beliefs expressed as stereotypes, rejection, and prejudice because of being overweight or obese (Puhl & Later, 2007). Children may face weight bias from multiple sources, including peers, teacher, health

care providers, and even parents. Children who are overweight might encounter verbal teasing (name calling, derogatory remarks), social exclusion (being ignored), and physical bullying (pushing, shoving). About one-third of overweight girls and one-quarter of overweight boys report being teased by peers at school.

Obese children who are victimized because of their weight are more vulnerable to depression, anxiety, lower self-esteem, and poor body image (Puhl & Later, 2007). With this awareness, childhood obesity prevention programs in schools and community settings to promote health in overweight and obese children must simultaneously protect them in the face of social stigmatization and its consequences.

Occupational Therapy Intervention

Traditional approaches to obesity have emphasized diet and exercise at the individual level; however, these strategies have had little impact on the growing increase of the obesity epidemic (Dehghan et al., 2005). Recent efforts call for broader attention to all of the physical, psychological, social, and spiritual dimensions of children's health in obesity prevention (O'Dea, 2005). In addition, because it is difficult to reduce excessive weight once it becomes established, prevention strategies need to begin while children are young and continue throughout the growing years. Strategies for intervention in children and youth can be embedded in several settings, including preschools and schools, after-school care, and community programs.

Framing Obesity Prevention Efforts: "First, Do No Harm."

According to O'Dea (2005), it is important to consider the possibility that some well-meaning prevention efforts may be more harmful than beneficial to children who are overweight. Child obesity prevention programs and untested health education messages have the potential to further stigmatize children who are overweight. The majority of children who are overweight are well aware of their body size and are at risk of developing a poor body image. Negatively focused health messages (e.g., that emphasize the undesirability of being overweight) may lead students to feel worse about themselves. Professionals must carefully consider how prevention messages are framed in order to avoid the potential psychosocial (e.g., poor self-esteem) and physical health (e.g., binge dieting) consequences that can result (Puhl & Later, 2007).

Take a Broader Focus: Promote Health Behaviors for All Children Regardless of Body Size

Prevention efforts that focus on health as both the primary motivator and desired outcome for positive lifestyle behaviors in all children may be more effective than those that focus on weight reduction in an isolated group (O'Dea, 2005). The "health at any size" movement has been successful in helping health professionals and people who are overweight focus on health improvement rather than weight status. Children of all weights should receive support from peers, adults, teachers, and parents to make healthy food choices and be physically active. Furthermore, in order to foster enjoyment in health behaviors, educators and health care providers need to remove blame from children who are overweight, provide education about weight bias to all adults and students, and implement policies that prohibit weight-based victimization (Puhl & Later, 2007).

Nutrition

A healthy diet has many benefits in addition to obesity prevention, including positive growth, physical development, brain development and cognition, and disease prevention (O'Dea, 2005). Occupational therapy practitioners can assess the availability of nutritious foods in children's schools and neighborhoods (Cahill & Suarez-Balcazar, 2009). Cooking activities that involve children in the planning and preparing of healthy snacks and meals can be embedded during the school day or in special after-school cooking groups. Attention to family habits and routines related to nutrition and mealtimes also may be beneficial. Working with school administration and staff to reduce vending machines that offer high-calorie foods and increasing nutritious lunches and snacks are strategies that support healthy eating habits for all children.

Physical Activity

Pressuring overweight children who are generally self-conscious of their bodies to participate in sports or physical activity inadvertently may reduce interest in ongoing participation (O'Dea, 2005). In contrast, engaging children in physical activities in which they are interested and that they enjoy is likely to foster positive feelings about being physically active and can have the added benefit of promoting social interaction and friendships.

There are numerous ways in which children and youth can be encouraged to be physically active throughout the day—doing an errand for the teacher, walking to visit a friend, helping weed the garden, or cleaning one's room. Exploring a range of physical activity options in addition to traditional exercise can be done individually or with groups of children and may include walking clubs, hiking, biking, or swimming, to name a few. If after-school clubs do not offer options for physical activity, occupational therapy practitioners might consider developing a program (Smallfield & Anderson, 2009).

Supporting school and community programs that offer noncompetitive sports teams can increase the likelihood that all children have opportunities to participate in and enjoy organized sports. In addition, children need to be taught about the mental health benefits of exercise. A growing body of research suggests that moderate regular exercise should be considered as a viable means of treating depression and anxiety and improving mental well-being in the general public (Fox, 1999).

Modifying Environments

A socioecologic, environmental model for increasing physical activity suggests that focusing on changing the physical environment, urban planning, and modes of transportation is likely to provide significant benefits in obesity prevention (O'Dea, 2005). Such a model emphasizes helping neighborhoods and communities develop safe, enjoyable, and inexpensive opportunities for physical activity, such as walking networks (designated safe walking paths and hiking trails), cycling networks (designated cycling routes and paths), public open spaces (safe parks and playgrounds), and safe and inexpensive recreation facilities (Dehghan et al., 2005).

Preventing Weight Bias and Promoting Weight Tolerance

There is increasing agreement that obesity prevention programs need to include strategies to prevent weight-based stigmatization in youth and promote weight tolerance (Puhl & Later, 2007). The adoption of school policies that prohibit weight-based teasing and victimization and the periodic assessment of bias to prevent unintentional stigmatization are also recommended. Occupational therapy practitioners need to become aware of their own biases related to overweight or obese children and youth and help foster school and community environments that are promote tolerance.

Prevention of Risky Teen Behaviors

Adolescents and college-age individuals take more risks than children or adults do, as indicated by statistics on automobile crashes, binge drinking, contraceptive use, and crime, but trying to understand why risk taking is more common during adolescence than during other periods of development has challenged psychologists for decades. (Steinberg, 2007, p. 55)

More than 90% of all American high school students have been educated in school about risks associated with teen sex, drug and substance abuse, and reckless driving, yet large proportions of them still have unsafe sex, binge drink, smoke cigarettes, and drive recklessly (Steinberg, 2004). According to developmental neuroscientists, a teen's inclination to engage in risky behavior is not due to lack of information or logical reasoning abilities (Steinberg, 2007). Instead, a lag in the development of psychosocial capacities (e.g., impulse control, delayed gratification, emotional regulation, resistance to peer influence) that regulates impulses contributes to adolescents' vulnerability for participation in risky behaviors.

These findings suggest that changing the contexts in which risky behavior occurs may be more successful than changing the way adolescents think about risk. For example, it is important for adults in home, school, and community settings to have a strong presence in teens' lives, to be vigilant about teen activities and behavior, and to be knowledgeable about a range of risky behaviors and associated symptoms.

Contextual factors have been linked to reductions in substance abuse and smoking. VanderWaal and colleagues (2005), for example, recommended that communities wishing to reduce smoking and drinking rates among adolescents should continue to provide supervised after-school activities for their youth. They found that adult-supervised after-school activities were significantly related to lower rates of cigarette smoking, alcohol use, and binge drinking. Encouraging all teens to participate in meaningful structured leisure activities during the after-school hours may, in fact, help reduce participation in risky behaviors (VanderWaal et al., 2005).

In a related way, the reduction of alcohol use may reduce the risk of suicide. Schilling and colleagues (2009) identified the use of alcohol while sad or depressed as associated with suicidal behavior in adolescents who may not engage in planning prior to an attempt.

In addition to fostering participation in meaningful activities and maintaining an adult presence in teens' lives, it is important for parents and professionals to be aware of signs associated with various risky behaviors. A risky behavior that many parents and health care professionals are unaware of is the "choking game," which involves self-strangulation or strangulation by another person with the hands or a noose to achieve a brief euphoric state caused by cerebral hypoxia. Although asphyxial games have been played by youth for generations, limited information about this activity has been reported in the medical literature (Andrew, Macnab, & Russell, 2009). The use of ligatures to induce asphyxia, as well as solo play, has made today's version of this phenomenon more dangerous, at times resulting in serious neurological injury or death (Toblin, Paulozzi, Gilchrist, & Russell, 2008).

Children who participate in this behavior clearly differ from those who commit suicide or engage in autoerotic activity. Those whose deaths have been reported in the media tend to be high-achieving and athletic youth who were not engaged in other risk-taking activities. Occupational therapy practitioners, along with parents, educators, coaches, and other health care providers, need to promote awareness of the dangers of this activity as well as associated symptoms. Warning signs that youth are participating in self-strangulation include frequent severe headaches; seizures; sudden vision loss; behavior change; bloodshot eyes; marks on the neck; disorientation after spending time alone; and ropes, scarves, and belts tied to bedroom furniture or doorknobs (Andrew et al., 2009; Toblin et al., 2008).

References

Accreditation Council for Occupational Therapy Education. (2012). 2011 Accreditation Council for Occupational Therapy Education (ACOTE®) standards. *American Journal of Occupational Therapy, 66,* S6–S74. http://dx.doi.org/10.5014/ajot.2012.66S6.

Agency for Healthcare Research and Quality, U.S. Preventive Services Task Force. (2009). *Standard recommendation language.* Retrieved February 14, 2009, from http://www.uspreventiveservice taskforce.uspstf.htm

Aldred, C., Green, J., & Adams, C. (2004). A new social communication intervention for children with autism: Pilot randomised controlled treatment study suggesting effectiveness. *Journal of Child Psychology and Psychiatry, 45,* 1420–1430. http://dx.doi.org/10.1111/j.1469-7610.2004.00338.x

American Occupational Therapy Association. (1979). Uniform terminology for occupational therapy. *Occupational Therapy News, 35,* 1-8.

American Occupational Therapy Association. (1989). Uniform terminology for occupational therapy (2nd ed.). *American Journal of Occupational Therapy, 48,* 1047-1054. http://dx.doi.org/10.5014/ajot.48.11.1047

American Occupational Therapy Association. (1994). Uniform terminology for occupational therapy (3rd ed.). *American Journal of Occupational Therapy, 48,* 1047–1054.

American Occupational Therapy Association. (2002). Occupational therapy practice framework: Domain and process. *American Journal of Occupational Therapy, 56,* 609-639. http://dx.doi.org/10.5014/ajot.56.6.609

American Occupational Therapy Association. (2006). *Transforming caseload to workload in school-based early intervention occupational therapy services.* Bethesda, MD: Author.

American Occupational Therapy Association (2008). Occupational therapy practice framework: Domain and process (2nd ed.). *American Journal of Occupational Therapy, 62,* 625-688. http://dx.doi.org/10.5014.ajot.62.6.625

American Occupational Therapy Association. (2009a). Guidelines for supervision, roles, and responsibilities during the delivery of occupational therapy services. *American Journal of Occupational Therapy, 63,* 797–803. http://dx.doi.org/10.5014/ajot.63.6.797

American Occupational Therapy Association. (2009b). Policy 1.44: Categories of occupational therapy personnel. In *Policy manual* (2011 ed., pp. 33–34). Bethesda, MD: Author.

American Occupational Therapy Association. (2010a). Occupational therapy services in the promotion of psychological and social aspects of mental health. *American Journal of Occupational Therapy, 64*(Suppl.), S78–S91. http://dx.doi.org/10.5014/ajot.2010.64S78

American Occupational Therapy Association. (2010b). Specialized knowledge and skills in mental health promotion, prevention, and intervention in occupational therapy practice. *American Journal of Occupational Therapy,*

64(Suppl.), S30–S43. http://dx.doi.org/10.5014/ajot.2010.64S30

American Occupational Therapy Association. (2013). Obesity and occupational therapy. *American Journal of Occupational Therapy, 67*(6 Suppl.).

American Psychiatric Association. (2000). *Diagnostic and statistical manual of mental disorders* (4th ed., text rev.). Washington, DC: Author.

Amish, P. L., Gesten, E. L., Smith, J. K., Clark, H. B., & Stark, C. (1988). Social problem-solving training for severely emotionally and behaviorally disturbed children. *Behavioral Disorders, 13,* 175–186.

Anderson, S. C., & Allen, L. R. (1985a). Effects of a leisure education program on activity involvement and social interaction of mentally retarded persons. *Adapted Physical Activity Quarterly, 2,* 107–116.

Anderson, S. C., & Allen, L. R. (1985b). Effects of a recreation therapy program on activity involvement and social interaction of mentally retarded persons. *Behaviour Research and Therapy, 23,* 473–477. http://dx.doi.org/10.1016/0005-7967(85)90176-7

Andrew, T. A., Macnab, A., & Russell, P. (2009). Update on "the choking game." *Journal of Pediatrics, 155,* 777–779. http://dx.doi.org/10.1016/j.jpeds.2009.06.043

Antia, S. D., & Kreimeyer, K. H. (1996). Social interaction and acceptance of deaf or hard-of-hearing children and their peers: A comparison of social-skills and familiarity-based interventions. *Volta Review, 98,* 157–180.

Aspy, R. & Grossman, B. (2007). *Underlying Characteristics Checklist—Classic Autism.* Overland Park, KS: AAPC Publishing.

Aspy, R., & Grossman, B. (2008). *Designing Comprehensive Interventions for Individuals with High-Functioning Autism and Asperger Syndrome: The Ziggurat Model.* Shawnee

Mission, KS: Autism Asperger Publishing Company (www.aapctextbooks.net).

Atkins, M. S., Hoagwood, K. E., Kutash, K., & Seidman, E. (2010). Toward the integration of education and mental health in schools. *Administration and Policy in Mental Health, 37,* 40–47. http://dx.doi.org/10.1007/s10488-010-0299-7

Attwood, T. (2002). *The profile of friendship skills in Asperger's syndrome.* Retrieved June 15, 2012, from http://www.tonyattwood.com.au/pdfs/attwood2.pdf

Baker, S. D., Lang, R., & O'Reilly, M. (2009). Review of video modeling with students with emotional and behavioral disorders. *Education and Treatment of Children, 32,* 403–420. http://dx.doi.org/10.1353/etc.0.0065

Barry, M. M., & Jenkins, R. (2007). *Implementing mental health promotion.* Edinburgh, UK: Churchill, Livingstone/Elsevier.

Batsche, G. M., & Porter, L. J. (2006). Bullying. In G. G. Bear & K. M. Minke (Eds.), *Children's needs III: Development, prevention, and intervention* (pp. 135–148). Bethesda, MD: National Association of School Psychologists.

Bauminger, N. (2007). Individual social-multimodal intervention for HFASD. *Journal of Autism and Developmental Disorders, 37,* 1593–1604. http://dx.doi.org/10.1007/s10803-006-0245-4

Bazyk, S. (2005). Creating occupation-based social skills groups in after-school care. *OT Practice, 11*(17), 13–18.

Bazyk, S., (2007). Addressing the mental health needs of children in schools. In L. Jackson (Ed.), *Occupational therapy services for children and youth under IDEA* (3rd ed., pp. 99–121). Bethesda, MD: AOTA Press.

Bazyk, S. (Ed.). (2011a). Enduring challenges and situational stressors during the school years: Risk reduction and competence enhancement. In S. Bazyk (Ed.), *Mental health promotion, prevention, and intervention with children and youth: A guiding framework for occupational therapy* (pp. 21–44). Bethesda, MD: AOTA Press.

Bazyk, S. (Ed.). (2011b). Occupational therapy process: A public health approach to promoting mental health in children and youth. In S. Bazyk (Ed.), *Mental health promotion, prevention, and intervention with children and youth* (pp. 21–44). Bethesda, MD: AOTA Press.

Bazyk, S. (Ed.). (2011c). *Mental health promotion, prevention, and intervention with children and youth: A guiding framework for occupational therapy.* Bethesda, MD: AOTA Press.

Bazyk, S., & Bazyk, J. (2009). Meaning of occupation-based groups for low income urban youth attending afterschool care. *American Journal of Occupational Therapy, 63,* 69–83. http://dx.doi.org/10.5014/ajot.63.1.69

Bazyk, S., & Bradenburger Shasby, S. (2011). Major approaches useful in addressing the mental health needs of children and youth: Minimizing risks, reducing symptoms, and building competencies. In S. Bazyk (Ed.), *Mental health promotion, prevention, and intervention with children and youth: A guiding framework for occupational therapy* (pp. 45–70). Bethesda, MD: AOTA Press.

Beets, M. W., Flay, B. R., Vuchinich, S., Snyder, F. J., Acock, A., Li, K., et al. (2009). Use of a social and character development program to prevent substance use, violent behaviors, and sexual activity among elementary-school students in Hawaii. *American Journal of Public Health, 99,* 1438–1445. http://dx.doi.org/10.2105/AJPH.2008.142919

Benavides, S., & Caballero, J. (2009). Astanga yoga for children and adolescents for weight management and psychological well being: An uncontrolled open pilot study. *Complementary Therapies in Clinical Practice, 15,* 110–114. http://dx.doi.org/10.1016/j.ctcp.2008.12.004

Berger, D. L., Silver, E. J., & Stein, R. E. (2009). Effects of yoga on inner-city children's well-

being: A pilot study. *Alternative Therapies in Health and Medicine, 15,* 36–42.

Bershad, C., & Blaber, C. (2011). *Realizing the promise of the whole-school approach to children's mental health: A practical guide for schools.* Washington, DC: Education Development Center.

Bhavnagri, N. P., & Samuels, B. G. (1996). Children's literature and activities promoting social cognition or peer relationships in preschoolers. *Early Childhood Research Quarterly, 11,* 307–331. http://dx.doi.org/10.1016/S088-2006(96)90010-1

Bierman, K. L., & Furman, W. (1984). The effects of social skills training and peer involvement on the social adjustment of preadolescents. *Child Development, 55,* 151–162. http://dx.doi.org/10.2307/1129841

Bierman, K. L., Miller, C. L., & Stabb, S. D. (1987). Improving the social behavior and peer acceptance of rejected boys: Effects of social skill training with instructions and prohibitions. *Journal of Consulting and Clinical Psychology, 55,* 194–200. http://dx.doi.org/10.1037/0022-006X.55.2.194

Birdee, G. S., Yeh, G. Y., Wayne, P. M., Phillips, R. S., Davis, R. B., & Gardiner, P. (2009). Clinical applications of yoga for the pediatric population: A systematic review. *Academic Pediatrics, 9,* 212–220. http://dx.doi.org/10.1016/j.acap.2009.04.002

Bloom, S. L. (1995). Creating sanctuary in the school. *Journal for a Just and Caring Education, 1,* 403–433.

Blum, R. W., & Rinehart, P. M. (1997). *Reducing the risk: Connections that make a difference in the lives of youth.* Minneapolis: University of Minnesota, Division of General Pediatrics and Adolescent Health.

Bosworth, K., Espelage, D., & DuBay, T. (1998). A computer-based violence prevention intervention for young adolescents: Pilot study. *Adolescence, 33,* 785–795.

Briggs-Gowan, M. J., & Carter, A. S. (2006). *BITSEA Brief Infant–Toddler Social and Emotional Assessment examiner's manual*. San Antonio, TX: Harcourt Assessment.

Brown, C., & Dunn, W. (2002). *Adolescent/Adult Sensory Profile®*. San Antonio, TX: Pearson.

Bruce, M. A., & Borg, B. (1993). *Psychosocial occupational therapy: Frames of reference for intervention*. Thorofare, NJ: Slack.

Butler, A. C., Chapman, J. E., Forman, E. M., & Beck, A. T. (2006). The empirical status of cognitive–behavioral therapy: A review of meta-analyses. *Clinical Psychology Review, 26*, 17–31. http://dx.doi.org/10.1016/j.cpr.2005.07.003

Cahill, S. M. (2007). A perspective on response to intervention. *School System Special Interest Section Quarterly, 14*(3), 1–4.

Cahill, S. M., & Suarez-Balcazar, Y. (2009). Promoting children's nutrition and fitness in the urban context. *American Journal of Occupational Therapy, 63*, 113–116. http://dx.doi.org/10.5014/ajot.63.1.113

Cardon, G. M., De Clercq, D. L. R., & DeBourdeaudhuij, L. M. M. (2002). Back education efficiency in elementary schoolchildren. *Spine, 27*, 299–305. http://dx.doi.org/10.1097/00007632-200202010-00020

Carr, E. G., Dunlap, G., Horner, R. H., Koegel, R. L., Turnbull, A., Sailor, W., et al (2002). Positive behavior support: Evolution of an applied science. *Journal of Positive Behavior Interventions, 4*(1), 4–16.

Carter, E. W., & Hughes, C. (2005). Increasing social interaction among adolescents with intellectual disabilities and their general education peers: Effective interventions. *Research and Practice for Persons With Severe Disabilities, 30*, 179–193. http://dx.doi.org/10.2511/rpsd.30.4.179

Cartledge, G. (2003). School-wide positive behavior management: A state improvement grant (SIG) partnership. *School-Wide Positive Behavior Management, 2*, 1–10.

Catalano, R. F., Hawkins, D., Berglund, M. L., Pollard, J. A., & Arthur, M. W. (2002). Prevention science and positive youth development: Competitive or cooperative frameworks? *Journal of Adolescent Health, 31*, 230–239. http://dx.doi.org/10.1016/S1054-139X(02)00496-2

Catterall, J. S., Dumais, S. A., & Hampden-Thomson, G. (2012). *The arts and achievement in at-risk youth: Findings from four longitudinal studies*. Washington DC: National Endowment for the Arts. Retrieved June 15, 2012, from http://www.nea.gov/research/Arts-At-Risk-Youth.pdf

Centers for Disease Control and Prevention. (2010). *Prevalence of overweight, obesity, and extreme obesity among adults: United States, trends 1960–1962 through 2007–2008*. Retrieved June 15, 2012, from http://www.cdc.gov/nchs/data/hestat/obesity_adult_07_08/obesity_adult_07_08.pdf

Centers for Disease Control and Prevention. (2012, March 30). Prevalence of autism spectrum disorders—Autism and Developmental Disabilities Monitoring Network, 14 sites, United States, 2008. *Morbidity and Mortality Weekly Report*, 1–19.

Champagne, T. (2008). *Sensory rooms in mental health*. Retrieved from http://www.ot-innovations.com/content/view/49/46/

Charlebois, P., Normandeau, S., Vitaro, F., & Berneche, F. (1999). Skills training for inattentive overactive, aggressive boys: Differential effects of contexts and delivery method. *Behavioral Disorders, 24*, 137–150.

Christian, B. J., & D'Auria, J. P. (2006). Life skills for children with cystic fibrosis: Effectiveness of an intervention. *Nursing Research, 55*, 300–307. http://dx.doi.org/10.1097/00006199-200609000-00002

Christner, R. W., Forrest, E., Morley, J., & Weinstein, E. (2007). Taking cognitive–behavior therapy to school: A school-based mental health approach. *Journal of Contemporary Psychotherapy, 37,* 175–183. http://dx.doi.org/10.1007/s10879-007-9052-2

Collaborative for Academic, Social, and Emotional Learning. (2009). *What is SEL? Skills and competencies.* Retrieved August 3, 2010, from www.casel.org/basics/skills.php

Conduct Problems Prevention Research Group. (2002). Evaluation of the first 3 years of the Fast Track Prevention Trial with children at high risk for adolescent conduct problems. *Journal of Abnormal Child Psychology, 30,* 19–35.

Conduct Problems Prevention Research Group. (2007). Fast track randomized controlled trial to prevent externalizing psychiatric disorders: Findings from Grades 3–9. *Journal of the American Academy of Child and Adolescent Psychiatry, 46,* 1250–1262. http://dx.doi.org/10.1097/chi.0b013e31813e5d39

Cook, C. R., Gresham, F. M., Kern, L., Barreras, R. B., Thornton, S., & Crews, S. D. (2008). Social skills training for secondary students with emotional and/or behavioral disorders: A review and analysis of the meta-analytic literature. *Journal of Emotional and Behavioral Disorders, 16,* 131–144. http://dx.doi.org/10.1177/1063426608314541

Coren, E., & Barlow, J. (2001). *Individual- and group-based parenting programmes for improving psychosocial outcomes for teenage parents and their children.* Cochrane Database of Systematic Reviews 2001, Issue 3, Article No. CD002964. http://dx.doi.org/10.1002/14651858.CD002964.

Coster, W. J., Deeney, T. A., Haltiwanger, J. T., & Haley, S. M. (1998). *School Function Assessment.* San Antonio, TX: Psychological Corporation/Therapy Skill Builders.

Cowen, E. (1991). In pursuit of wellness. *American Psychologist, 46,* 404–408. http://dx.doi.org/10.1037/0003-066X.46.4.404

Crabtree, L., & Delaney, J. V. (2011). Autism: Promoting social participation and mental health. In S. Bazyk (Ed.), *Mental health promotion, prevention, and intervention with children and youth: A guiding framework for occupational therapy* (pp. 163–187). Bethesda, MD: AOTA Press.

Csapo, M. (1986). Social skills training with neglected and rejected children. *Journal of Special Education, 10,* 321–338.

Csikszentmihalyi, M. (1993). Activity and happiness: Towards a science of occupation. *Occupational Science, 1,* 38–42. http://dx.doi.org/10.1080/14427591.1993.9686377

Davidson, D. A. (2005). Psychosocial issues affecting social participation. In J. Case-Smith (Ed.), *Occupational therapy for children* (5th ed., pp. 449–480). St. Louis, MO: Elsevier/Mosby.

Daykin, N., Orme, J., Evans, D., Salmon, D., McEachran, M., & Brain, S. (2008). The impact of participation in performing arts on adolescent health and behavior: A systematic review of the literature. *Journal of Health Psychology, 13,* 251–264. http://dx.doi.org/10.1177/1359105307086699

De, S., Small, J., & Baur, L. A., (2008). Overweight and obesity among children with developmental disabilities. *Journal of Intellectual and Developmental Disability, 33,* 43–47. http://dx.doi.org/1080/13668250701875137

Dehghan, M., Akhtar-Danesh, N., & Merchant, A. T. (2005). Childhood obesity, prevalence and prevention. *Nutrition Journal, 4,* 1–8. http://dx.doi.org/10.1186/1475-2891-4-1

DeMar, J. (1997). A school-based group intervention to strengthen personal and social competencies in latency-age children. *Social Work in Education, 19,* 219–230.

Demir, M., & Weitekamp, L. A. (2007). I am so happy cause today I found my friend: Friendship and personality as predictors of happiness. *Journal of Happiness Studies, 8,* 181–211. http://dx.doi.org/1007/s10902-006-9012-7

Demir, M., Zdemir, M., & Weitekamp, L. A. (2007). Looking to happy tomorrows with friends: Best and close friendships as they predict happiness. *Journal of Happiness Studies, 8,* 243–271. http://dx.doi.org/10.1007/s10902-006-9012-7

Diener, E. (2000). Subjective well-being: The science of happiness and a proposal for a national index. *American Psychologist, 55,* 34–43. http://dx.doi.org/10.1037/0003-066X.55.1.34

Dobson, D. J. G., McDougall, G., Busheikin, J., & Aldous, J. (1995). Effects of social skills training and social milieu treatment on symptoms of schizophrenia. *Psychiatric Services, 46,* 376–380.

Dolgin, M. J., Somer, E., Zaidel, N., & Zaizov, R. (1997). A structured group intervention for siblings of children with cancer. *Journal of Child and Adolescent Group Therapy, 7,* 3–18. http://dx.doi.org/10.1007/BF02548945

Downing, D. (2011). Occupational therapy for youth at risk of psychosis and those with identified mental illness. In S. Bazyk (Ed.), *Mental health promotion, prevention, and intervention with children and youth: A guiding framework for occupational therapy* (pp. 141–161). Bethesda, MD: AOTA Press.

Drysdale, J., Casey, J., & Porter-Armstrong, A. (2008). Effectiveness of training on the community skills of children with intellectual disabilities. *Scandinavian Journal of Occupational Therapy, 15,* 247–255. http://dx.doi.org/10.1080/11038120802456136

Dubow, E. F., Huesmann, L. R., & Eron, L. D. (1987). Mitigating aggression and promoting prosocial behavior in aggressive elementary schoolboys. *Behaviour Research and Therapy, 25,* 527–531. http://dx.doi.org/10.1016/0005-7967(87)90061-1

Duffy, B., & Fuller, R. (2000). Role of music therapy in social skills development in children with moderate intellectual disability. *Journal of*

Applied Research in Intellectual Disabilities, 13, 77–89. http://dx.doi.org/10.1046/j.1468-3148.2000.00011.x

Duncan, B. B., Forness, S. R., & Harsough, C. (1995). Students identified as seriously emotionally disturbed in school-based day treatment: Cognitive, psychiatric, and special educational characteristics. *Behavioral Disorders, 20,* 238–252.

Dunn, W. (1999). *The Sensory Profile Manual.* San Antonio: Psychological Corporation.

Dunn, W. (2000). *Best practice occupational therapy: In community service with children and families.* Thorofare, NJ: Slack.

Dunn, W. (2007). Supporting children to participate successfully in everyday life by using sensory processing knowledge. *Infants and Young Children, 20,* 84–101. http://dx.doi.org/10.1097/01.IYC.0000264477.05076.5d

Dunn, W., Brown, C., & Youngstrom, M. J. (2003). Ecological model of occupation. In P. Kramer, J. Hinojosa, & C. B. Royeen (Eds.), *Perspectives on human occupation: Participation in life* (pp. 222–263). Philadelphia: Lippincott Williams & Wilkins.

Durlak, J. A., Weissberg, R. P., Dymnicki, A. B., Taylor, R. D., & Schellinger, K. B. (2011). The impact of enhancing students' social and emotional learning: A meta-analysis of school-based universal interventions. *Child Development, 82,* 405–432. http://dx.doi.org/10.1111/j.1467-8624.2010.01564.x

Durlak, J. A., Weissberg, R. P., & Pachan, M. (2010). A meta-analysis of after-school programs that seek to promote personal and social skills in children and adolescents. *American Journal of Community Psychology, 45,* 294–309. http://dx/doi.org/10.1007/s10464-010-9300-6

Dworkin, J. (2003). Adolescents' accounts of growth experiences in youth activities. *Journal of Youth and Adolescence, 32,* 17–26. http://dx.doi.org/10.1023/A:1021076222321

Dworkin, J. B., Larson, R., & Hansen, D. (2003). Adolescents' accounts of growth experiences in youth activities. *Journal of Youth and Adolescence, 32*, 17–26. http://dx.doi.org/10.1023/A:1021076 22321

Dwyer, G., Baur, L., Higgs, J., & Hardy, L. (2009). Promoting children's health and well-being: Broadening the therapy perspective. *Physical and Occupational Therapy in Pediatrics, 29*, 27–43. http://dx.doi.org/10.1080/01942630802574825

Ebbeck, V., & Gibbons, S. L. (1998). The effect of a team building program on the self-conceptions of Grade 6 and 7 physical education students. *Journal of Sport and Exercise Psychology, 20*, 300–310.

Eccles, J. S., & Gootman, J. A. (Eds.). (2002). *Community programs to promote youth development*. Washington, DC: National Academy Press.

Education for All Handicapped Children Act of 1975, Pub. L. 94–142, 20 U.S.C. § 1400 *et seq.*

Elias, M. J., Zins, J. E., Weissberg, K. S., Frey, K. S., Greenberg, M. T., Haynes, N. M., et al. (Eds.). (1997). *Promoting social and emotional learning: Guidelines for educators*. Alexandria, VA: Association for Supervision and Curriculum.

Emerson, E. (2009). Overweight and obesity in 3- and 5-year-old children with and without developmental delay. *Public Health, 123*, 130–133. http://dx.doi.org/10.1016/j.puhe.2008.10.020

Emmer, E. T., & Stough, L. M. (2001). Classroom management: A critical part of educational psychology, with implications for teacher education. *Educational Psychologist, 36*, 103–112. http://dx.doi.org/10.1207/S15326985EP3602_5

Epp, K. M. (2008). Outcome-based evaluation of a social skills program using art therapy and group therapy for children on the autism spectrum. *Children and Schools, 30*, 27–36. http://dx.doi.org/10.1093/cs/30.1.27

Espelage, D. L., & Swearer, S. M. (2003). Research on school bullying and victimization: What have we learned and where do we go from here? *School Psychology Review, 32*, 365–383.

Fantuzzo, J., Sutton-Smith, B., Atkins, M., Meyers, R., Stevenson, H., Coolahan, K., et al. (1996). Community-based resilient peer treatment of withdrawn maltreated preschool children. *Journal of Consulting and Clinical Psychology, 64,* 1377–1386. http://dx.doi.org/10.1037/0022-006X.64.5.1377

Felitti, V. J., Anda, R. F., Nordenberg, D., Williamson, D. F., Spitz, A. M., Edwards, V., et al. (1998). Relationship of childhood abuse and household dysfunction to many of the leading causes of death in adults: The Adverse Childhood Experiences (ACE) Study. *American Journal of Preventive Medicine, 14*, 245–258. http://dx.doi.org/10.1061/S0749-3797(98)00017-8

Fisher, A. G., & Bray Jones, K. (2010). *Assessment of Motor and Process Skills. Vol 2: User manual* (7th ed.). Fort Collins, CO: Three Star Press.

Forness, S. R. (2003). Barriers to evidence-based treatment: Developmental psychopathology and the interdisciplinary disconnect in school mental health practice. *Journal of School Psychology, 41*, 61–67. http://dx.doi.org/10.1016/S0022-4405(02)00144-9

Forness, S. R., Kavale, K. A., MacMillan, D. L., Asarnow, J. R., & Duncan, B. B. (1996). Early detection and prevention of emotional or behavioral disorders: Developmental aspects of systems of care. *Behavioral Disorders, 21*, 226–240.

Fox, K. R. (1999). The influence of physical activity on mental well-being. *Public Health Nutrition, 2*, 411–418. http://dx.doi.org/10.1017/S1368980099000567

Frankel, F., Myatt, R., Cantwell, D., & Feinberg, D. (1997). Parent-assisted transfer of children's social skills training: Effects on children with and without attention-deficit hyperactivity disorder. *Journal of the American Academy of Child and Adolescent Psychology, 36,* 1056–1064. http://dx.doi.org/10.1097/00004583-199708000-00013

Freeman, R., Eber, L., Anderson, C., Irvin, L., Bounds, M., Dunlap, G., et al. (2006). Building inclusive school cultures using school-wide positive behavior support: Designing effective individual support systems for students with significant disabilities. *Research and Practice for Persons With Severe Disabilities, 31,* 4–17. http://dx.doi.org/10.2511/rpsd.31.1.4

Frolek Clark, G., & Kingsley, K. (2013). *Occupational therapy practice guidelines for early childhood: Birth through 5 years.* Bethesda, MD: AOTA Press.

Galantino, M. L., Galbavy, R., & Quinn, L. (2008). Therapeutic effects of yoga for children: A systematic review of the literature. *Pediatric Physical Therapy, 20,* 66–80. http://dx.doi.org/10.1097/PEP.0b013e31815f1208

Gangl, M. L. (1987). The effectiveness of an occupational therapy program for chemically dependent adolescents. *Occupational Therapy in Mental Health, 7,* 67–88. http://dx.doi.org/10.1300/J004v07n02_06

Gebert, N., Hummelink, J., Konning, J., Staab, D., Schmidt, S., Szczepanski, R., et al. (1998). Efficacy of self-management program for childhood asthma—A prospective study. *Patient Education and Counseling, 35,* 213–220. http://dx.doi.org/10.1016/S0738-3991(98)00061-5

Geldhof, E., Cardon, G., De Bourdeaudhuij, I., & De Clercq, D. (2007). Back posture education in elementary schoolchildren: A 2-year follow-up study. *European Spine Journal, 16,* 841–850. http://dx/doi.org/10.1007/s00586-006-0227-4

Gencoz, F. (1997). The effects of basketball training on the maladaptive behaviors of trainable mentally retarded children. *Research in Developmental Disabilities, 18,* 1–10. http://dx.doi.org/10.1016/S0891-4222(96)00029-7

Ginsburg, G. S., & Kingery, J. N. (2007). Evidence-based practice for childhood anxiety disorders. *Journal of Contemporary Psychotherapy, 37,* 123–132. http://dx.doi.org/10.1007/s10879-007-9047-z

Girolametto, L. E. (1988). Improving the social-conversational skills of developmentally delayed children: An intervention study. *Journal of Speech and Hearing Disorders, 53,* 156–167.

Gold, C., Wigram, T., & Elefant, C. (2006). *Music therapy for autistic spectrum disorder.* Cochrane Database of Systematic Reviews 2006, Issue 2, Article No. CD004381. http://dx.doi.org/10.1002/14651858.CD004381.pub2

Goleman, D. (1995). *Emotional intelligence: Why it can matter more than IQ.* New York: Bantam Books.

Gowen, L. K., & Walker, J. S. (2009). Youth empowerment and participation in mental health care. *FOCAL POiNT: Research, Policy, and Practice in Children's Mental Health, 23*(2), 3–5.

Graham, F., Rodger, S., & Ziviani, J. (2009). Coaching parents to enable children's participation: An approach for working with parents and their children. *Australian Occupational Therapy Journal, 56,* 16–23. http://dx.doi.org/10.1111/j.1440-1630.2008.00736.x

Greenberg, M. T., Weissberg, R. P., O'Brian, M., Zins, J. E., Fredericks, L., Resnik, H., et al. (2003). Enhancing school-based prevention and youth development through coordinated social, emotional, and academic learning. *American Psychologist, 58,* 466–474. http://dx.doi.org/10.1037/0003-066X.58.6-7.466

Gresham, F., & Elliott, S. (1990). *The Social Skills Rating System.* Circle Pines, MN: American Guidance Service.

Griffiths, K. M., Christensen, H., & Jorm, A. F. (2009). Mental health literacy as a function of remoteness of residence: An Australian national study. *BMC Public Health, 9,* 1–20. Retrieved June 15, 2012, from http://www.biomedcentral.com/1471-2458/9/92

Grizenko, N., Papineau, D., & Sayegh, L. (1993a). A comparison of day treatment and outpatient treatment for children with disruptive behavior. *Canadian Journal of Psychiatry, 38,* 432–435.

Grizenko, N., Papineau, D., & Sayegh, L. (1993b). Effectiveness of a multimodal day treatment program for children with disruptive behavior problems. *Journal of the American Academy of Child and Adolescent Psychiatry, 32,* 127–134. http://dx.doi.org/10.1097/00004583-199301000-00019

Guy, S., Ratzki-Leewing, A., & Gwadry-Sridhar, F. (2011). Moving beyond the stigma: Systematic review of video games and their potential to combat obesity. *International Journal of Hypertension, 2011,* 1–13. http://dx.doi.org/10.4061/2011/179124

Hansen, D., Larson, R., & Dworkin, J. B. (2003). What adolescents learn in organized youth activities: A survey of self-reported developmental experiences. *Journal of Research on Adolescence, 13,* 25–55. http://dx.doi.org/10.1111/1532-7795.1301006

Heinrich, R. H. (2003). A whole-school approach to bullying: Special considerations for children with exceptionalities. *Intervention in School and Clinic, 38,* 195–204. http://dx.doi.org/10.1177/105345120303800401

Henry, D. (2001). *The tool chest: For teachers, parents and students.* Glendale, AZ: Henry OT.

Hepler, J. B., & Rose, S. F. (1988). Evaluation of a multi-component group approach for improving the social skills of elementary school children. *Journal of Social Service Research, 11*(4), 1–18. http://dx.doi.org/10.1300/J079v11n04_01

Hernandez-Guzman, L., Gonzalez, S., & Lopez, F. (2002). Effect of guided imagery on children's social performance. *Behavioural and Cognitive Psychotherapy, 30,* 471–483. http://dx.doi.org/10.1017/S1352465802004083

Hoagwood, K., & Johnson, J. (2003). School psychology: A public health framework: I. From evidence-based practices to evidence-based policies. *Journal of School Psychology, 41,* 3–21. http://dx.doi.org/10.1016/S0022-4405(02)00141-3

Hoffman, O. R., Hemmingsson, H., & Kielhofner, G. (2000). *The School Setting Interview: A user's manual.* Chicago: University of Illinois, Department of Occupational Therapy.

Ikiugu, M., & Ciaravino, E. A. (2006). Assisting adolescents experiencing emotional and behavioral difficulties (EBD) transition to adulthood. *International Journal of Psychosocial Rehabilitation, 10,* 57–78.

Individuals with Disabilities Education Act of 1997, Pub. L. 105–117, 20 U.S.C. §1400 *et seq.*

Individuals With Disabilities Education Improvement Act of 2004, Pub. L. 108–446, 20 U.S.C. § 1400 *et seq.*

Institute of Medicine, Committee for the Study of the Future of Public Health, Division of Health Care Services. (1988). *The future of public health.* Washington, DC: National Academies Press.

Ison, M. S. (2001). Training in social skills: An alternative technique for handling disruptive child behavior. *Psychological Reports, 88,* 903–911. http://dx.doi.org/10.2466/pr0.2001.88.3.703

Jackson, L. L., & Arbesman, M. (2005). *Occupational therapy practice guidelines for children with behavioral and psychosocial needs.* Bethesda, MD: AOTA Press.

Jackson, M. F., & Marziller, J. S. (1983). An investigation of the treatment of adolescent social difficulty in a community-based setting. *Behavioural Psychotherapy, 11,* 302–319. http://dx.doi.org/10.1017/S0141347300008612

Jeffree, D. M., & Cheseldine, S. E. (1984). Programmed leisure intervention and the interaction patterns of severely mentally retarded adolescents: A pilot study. *Journal of Mental Deficiency, 88,* 619–624.

Jenson, J. M., & Dieterich, W. A. (2007). Effects of a skills-based prevention program on bullying and bully victimization among elementary school children. *Prevention Science, 8,* 285–296. http://dx.doi.org/10.1007/s11121-007-0076-3

Jones, M. B., & Offord, D. R. (1989). Reeducation of antisocial behavior in poor children by nonschool skill development. *Journal of Child Psychiatry, 30,* 737–750. http://dx.doi.org/10.1111/j.1469-7610.1989.tb00786.x

Jorm, A. F. (2012). Mental health literacy: Empowering the community to take action for better mental health. *American Psychologist, 67,* 231–243.

Jorm, A. F., Korten, A. E., Jacomb, P. A., Christensen, H., Rodgers, B., & Pollitt, P. (1997). "Mental health literacy": A survey of the public's ability to recognize mental disorders and their beliefs about the effectiveness of treatment. *Medical Journal of Australia, 166,* 182–186.

Kamps, D. M., Tankersley, M., & Ellis, C. (2000). Social skills interventions for young at-risk students: A 2-year follow-up study. *Behavioral Disorders, 25,* 310–324.

Kannenberg, K., & Greene, S. (2003, June 2). Infusing occupation into practice: Valuing and supporting the psychosocial foundation of occupation. *OT Practice,* pp. CE1–CE8.

Kazdin, A. E., Bass, D., Siegel, T., & Thomas, C. (1989). Cognitive–behavioral therapy and relationship therapy in the treatment of children referred for antisocial behavior. *Journal of Consulting and Clinical Psychology, 57,* 522–535. http://dx.doi.org/10.1037/0022-006X.57.4.522

Kessler, R. C., Berglund, P., Demler, O., Jin, R., Merinkangas, K. R., & Walters, E. E. (2005). Lifetime prevalence and age-of-onset distributions of *DSM–IV* disorders in the National Comorbidity Survey Replication. *Archives of General Psychiatry, 62,* 593–602. http://dx.doi.org/10.1001/archpsyc.62.6.593

Keyes, C. L. (2007). Promoting and protecting mental health as flourishing: A complementary strategy for improving national mental health. *American Psychologist, 62,* 95–108. http://dx.doi.org/10.1037/0003-066X.62.2.95

Kim, J., Wigram, T., & Gold, C. (2008). The effects of improvisational music therapy on joint attention behaviors in autistic children: A randomized controlled study. *Journal of Autism and Developmental Disorders, 38,* 1758–1766. http://dx.doi.org/10.1007/s10803-008-0566-6

King, G., Law, M., King, S., Hurley, P., Hanna, S. Kertoy, M., et al. (2004). *Children's Assessment of Participation and Enjoyment (CAPE) and Preferences for Activities of Children (PAC).* San Antonio, TX: Harcourt Assessment.

Kingsnorth, S., Healy, H., & MacArthur, C. (2007). Preparing for adulthood: A systematic review of life skill programs for youth with physical disabilities. *Journal of Adolescent Health, 41,* 323–332. http://dx.doi.org/10.1016/j.jadohealth.2007.06.007

Kinnevy, S. C., Healy, B. P., Pollio, D. E., & North, C. S. (1999). BicycleWORKS: Task-centered group work with high-risk youth. *Social Work With Groups, 22,* 33–47. http://dx.doi.org/10.1300/J009v22n01_03

Kleiber, D. (1999). *Leisure experience and human development: A dialectical approach.* New York: Basic Books.

Koegel, R. L., Dyer, K., & Bell, L. K. (1987). The influence of child-preferred activities on autistic children's social behavior. *Journal of Applied Behavior Analysis, 20,* 243–252. http://dx.doi.org/10.1901/jaba.1987.20-243

Koller, J. R., & Bertel, J. M. (2006). Responding to today's mental health needs of children, families and schools: Revisiting the preservice training and preparation of school-based personnel. *Education and Treatment of Children, 29,* 197–217.

Koppelman, J. (2004). *Children with mental disorders: Making sense of their needs and systems that help them* (NHPF Issue Brief No. 799). Washington, DC: National Health Policy Forum.

Kraag, G., Zeegers, M. P., Kok, G., Hosman, C., & Abu-Saad, H. H. (2006). School programs targeting stress management in children and adolescents: A meta-analysis. *Journal of School Psychology, 44,* 440–472. http://dx.doi.org/10.1016/j.jsp.2000.07.001

Kroeger, K. A., Schultz, J. R., & Newson, C. (2007). A comparison of two group-delivered social skills programs for young children with autism. *Journal of Autism and Developmental Disorders, 37,* 808–817. http://dx.doi.org/10.1007/s10803-006-0207-x

Kusche, C. A., & Greenberg, M. T. (1994). *The PATHS (Promoting Alternative Thinking Strategies) curriculum.* Seattle, WA: Developmental Research and Programs.

Kutash, K., Duchnowski, A. J., & Lynn, N. (2006). *School-based mental health: An empirical guide for decision-makers.* Tampa: University of South Florida Press.

Kutnick, P. J., & Brees, P. (1982). The development of co-operation: Explorations on cognitive and moral competence and social authority. *British Journal of Educational Psychology, 52,* 361–365. http://dx.doi.org/10.1111/j.2044-8279.1982.tb02522.x

Lamb, S. J., Bibby, P. A., & Wood, D. J. (1997). Promoting the communication skills of children with moderate learning difficulties. *Child Language Teaching and Therapy, 13,* 261–278. http://dx.doi.org/10.1177/026565909701300304

Larson, R. W. (2000). Toward a psychology of positive youth development. *American Psychologist, 55,* 170–183. http://dx.doi.org/10.1037/0003-066X.55.1.170

Laugeson, E. A., Frankel, F., Mogil, C., & Dillon, A. R. (2009). Parent-assisted social skills training to improve friendships in teens with autism spectrum disorders. *Journal of Autism and Developmental Disorders, 39,* 596–606. http://dx.doi.org/10.1007/s10803-008-0664-5

Law, M. Baptiste, S., Carswell, A., McColl, M. A., Polatajko, H., & Pollock, N. (2005). *The Canadian Performance Measure* (4th ed.). Ottawa, ON: Canadian Association of Occupational Therapy.

Law, M., & Baum, C. (1998). Evidence-based occupational therapy. *Canadian Journal of Occupational Therapy, 65,* 131–135.

Law, M., Cooper, B., Strong, S., Stewart, D., Rigby, P., & Letts, L. (1996). The person–environment-occupation model: A transactive approach to occupational therapy performance. *Canadian Journal of Occupational Therapy, 63,* 9–23.

LeBuffe, P., Shapiro, V., & Naglieri, J. (2009). *Devereux Student Strengths Assessment.* Lewisville, NC: Kaplan.

Lee, S.-H., Simpson, R. L., & Shogren, K. A. (2007). Effects and implications of self-management for students with autism: A meta-analysis. *Focus on Autism and Other Developmental Disabilities, 22,* 2–13. http://dx.doi.org/10.1177/10883576070220010101

Lefebvre-Pinard, M., & Reid, L. (1980). A comparison of three methods of training communication skills: Social conflict, modeling, and conflict-modeling. *Child Development, 51,* 179–187. http://dx.doi.org/10.2307/1129605

LeGoff, D. B. (2004). Use of LEGO® as a therapeutic medium for improving social competence. *Journal of Autism and Developmental Disorders, 34,* 557–571. http://dx.doi.org/10.1007/s10803-004-2550-0

LeGoff, D. B., & Sherman, M. (2006). Long-term outcome of social skills intervention based in interactive LEGO® play. *Autism, 1,* 317–329. http://dx.doi.org/10.1177/1362361306064403

Lochman, J. E., Haynes, S. M., & Dobson, E. G. (1981). Psychosocial effects of an intensive summer communication program for cleft palate children. *Child Psychiatry and Human Development, 12,* 54–62. http://dx.doi.org/10.1007/BF00706674

Lochman, J. E., & Wells, K. C. (2002). The Coping Power program at the middle-school transition: Universal and indicated prevention effects. *Psychology of Addictive Behaviors, 16,* S40–S54. http://dx.doi.org/10.1037/0893-164X.16.4S.S40

Lochman, J. E., & Wells, K. C. (2003). Effectiveness of the Coping Power program and of classroom intervention with aggressive children: Outcomes at a 1-year follow-up. *Behavior Therapy, 34,* 493–515. http://dx.doi.org/10.1016/S0005-7894(03)80032-1

Lochman, J. E., & Wells, K. C. (2004). The Coping Power program for preadolescent aggressive boys and their parents: Outcome effects at the 1-year follow-up. *Journal of Consulting and Clinical Psychology, 72,* 571–578. http://dx.doi.org/10.1037/0022-006X.72.4.571

Lopata, C., Thomeer, M. L., Volker, M. A., Nida, R. E., & Lee, G. K. (2008). Effectiveness of a manualized summer social treatment program for high-functioning children with autism spectrum disorders. *Journal of Autism and Devel-opmental Disorders, 38,* 890–904. http://dx.doi.org/10.1007/s10803-007-0460-7

Lopez, M., Forness, S. R., MacMillan, D. L., Bocian, K., & Gresham, F. M. (1996). Children with attention deficit hyperactivity disorder and emotional or behavioral disorders in the primary grades: Inappropriate placement in the learning disability category. *Educational Treatment of Children, 19,* 286–299.

Lougher, L. (2001). *Occupational therapy for children and adolescent mental health.* Edinburgh, UK: Churchill Livingstone.

Lowenstein, L. F. (1982). The treatment of extreme shyness in maladjusted children by implosive counseling and conditioning approaches. *Acta Psychiatrica Scandinavica, 66,* 173–189. http://dx.doi.org/10.1111/j.1600-0447.1982.tb00926.x

Machalicek, W., O'Reilly, M. F., Beretvas, N., Sigafoos, J., & Lancioni, G. E. (2007). A review of interventions to reduce challenging behavior in school setting for students with autism spectrum disorders. *Research in Autism Spectrum Disorders, 1,* 229–246. http://dx.doi.org/10.1080/13668250701589280

Mackay, T., Knott, F., & Dunlop, A.-W. (2007). Developing social interaction and understanding in individuals with autism spectrum disorder: A groupwork intervention. *Journal of Intellectual and Developmental Disability, 32,* 279–290. http://dx.doi.org/10.1080/13668250701689280

Mahoney, J. L., Harris, A. L., & Eccles, J. S. (2008). *The over-scheduling myth.* Retrieved June 15, 2012, from http://www.childtrends.org/Files//Child_Trends-2008_02_27_Myth.pdf

Mahoney, J. L., Larson, R. W., Eccles, J. S., & Lord, H. (2005). Organized activities as development contexts for children and adolescents. In J. Mahoney, R. Larson, & J. Eccles (Eds.), *Organized activities as contexts of development: Extracurricular activities, after-school and com-*

munity programs (pp. 3–23). Mahwah, NJ: Erlbaum.

Mahoney, J. L., & Stattin, H. (2000). Leisure activities and adolescent antisocial behavior: The role of structure and social context. *Journal of Adolescence, 23,* 113–127. http://dx.doi.org/10.1006/jado.2000.0302

Manly, T., Robertson, I. H., Anderson, V., & Nimmo-Smith, I. (1998). *The Test of Everyday Attention for Children (TEA-Ch).* San Antonio, TX: Pearson

Masia-Warner, C., Nangle, D. W., & Hansen, D. J. (2006). Bringing evidence-based child mental health services to the schools: General issues and specific populations. *Education and Treatment of Children, 29,* 165–172.

Masten, A. S. (2006). Developmental psychology: Pathways to the future. *International Journal of Behavioral Development, 30,* 47–54. http://dx.doi.org/10.1177/0165025406059974

Masten, A. S., Roisman, G. I., Long, J. D., Burt, K. B., Obradovic, J., Riley, J. R., et al. (2005). Developmental cascades: Linking academic achievement and externalizing and internalizing symptoms over 20 years. *Developmental Psychology, 41,* 733–746. http://dx.doi.org/10.1037/0012-1649.41.5.733

McLaughlin, M. (2000). *Community counts: How youth organizations matter for youth development.* Washington, DC: Public Education Network.

McMahon, S. D., Washburn, J., Felix, E. D., Yakin, J., & Childrey, G. (2000). Violence prevention: Program effects on urban preschool and kindergarten children. *Applied and Preventative Psychology, 9,* 271–281. http://dx.doi.org/10.1016/S0092-1849(00)80004-9

McNeil, D. A., Wilson, B. N., Siever, J. E., Ronca, M., & Mah, J. K. (2009). Connecting children to recreational activities: Results of a cluster randomized trial. *American Journal of Health Promotion, 23,* 376–387. http://dx.doi.org/10.4278/ajhp.071010107

McPherson, A. C., Glazebrook, C., Forster, D., James, C., & Smyth, A. (2006). A randomized, controlled trial of an interactive educational computer package for children with asthma. *Pediatrics, 117,* 1046–1054. http://dx.doi.org/10.1542/peds.2005-0666

Mevarech, Z. R., & Kramarski, B. (1993). Vygotsky and Papert: Social–cognitive interactions within Logo environments. *British Journal of Educational Psychology, 63,* 96–109. http://dx.doi.org/10.1111/j.2044-8279.1993.tb01044.x

Miles, J., Espiritu, R. C., Horen, N., Sebian, J., & Waetzig, E. (2010). *A public health approach to children's mental health: A conceptual framework.* Washington, DC: Georgetown University Center for Child and Human Development, National Technical Assistance Center for Children's Mental Health.

Miller Kuhaneck, H., Henry, D., Glennon, T., Parham, L. D., & Ecker, C. (2008). *The Sensory Processing Measure.* Los Angeles: Western Psychological Services.

Minnesota Association for Children's Mental Health. (2009). *Mental Health Fact Sheets—Fact Sheets for the Classroom.* Retrieved June 15, 2012, from www.schoolmentalhealth.org/resources/educ/macmh/macmh.html

Missiuna, C., Pollock, N., & Law, M. (2004). *Perceived efficacy and goal setting system (PEGS).* San Antonio, TX: Psychological Corporation.

Moherek Sopko, K. (2006). *School mental health services in the United States.* Retrieved June 15, 2012, from http://www.projectforum.org/docs/SchoolMentalHealthServicesintheUS.pdf

Molineux, M. L., & Whiteford, G. (1999). Prisons: From occupational deprivation to occupational enrichment. *Journal of Occupational Science, 6,*

124–130. http://dx.doi.org/10.1080/14427591.199
9.9686457

Monga, S., Young, A., & Owens, M. (2009). Evaluating a cognitive–behavioral therapy group program for anxious five- to seven-year-old children: A pilot study. *Depression and Anxiety, 26,* 243–250. http://dx.doi.org/10.1002/da.20551

Moody, K. A., Childs, J. C., & Sepples, S. B. (2003). Intervening with at-risk youth: Evaluation of the youth empowerment and support program. *Pediatric Nursing, 29,* 263–270.

Morris, T. L., Messer, S. C., & Gross, A. M. (1995). Enhancement of the social interaction and status of neglected children: A peer-pairing approach. *Journal of Clinical Child Psychology, 24,* 11–20. http://dx.doi.org/10.1207/s1537442jccp2401_2

Mrazek, P. J., & Haggerty, R J. (Eds.). (1994). *Reducing risks for mental disorders.* Washington, DC: National Academies Press.

Mu, K., & Gabriel, L. (2001). Comprehensive behavior support: Strategies to cope with severe challenging behavior. *OT Practice, 6,* 12–17.

Mulcahy, G. A., & Schachter, J. G. (1982). Cognitive self-modeling, conventional group counseling, and change in interpersonal skills. *Genetic Psychology Monographs, 106,* 117–175.

Nansel, T. R., Overpeck, M., Pilla, R. S., Ruan, W. J., Simons-Morton, B., & Scheidt, P. (2001). Bullying behaviors among U.S. youth: Prevalence and associations with psychosocial adjustment. *Journal of the American Medical Association, 285,* 2094–2100. http://dx.doi.org/10.1011/jama.285.16.2094

National Research Council, & Institute of Medicine. (2009). *Preventing mental, emotional, and behavioral disorders among young people: Progress and possibilities.* Washington, DC: National Academies Press.

National Survey on Drug Use and Health. (2005). *Youth prevention-related measures.* Retrieved June 15, 2012, from http://www.oas.samhsa.gov/nsduh/2k4nsduh/2k4results/2k4results.htm#ch6

No Child Left Behind Act of 2001, Pub. L. 107–110, 115 Stat. 1425 (2002).

O'Connell, M. E., Boar, T., & Warner, K. E. (2009) Using a developmental framework to guide prevention and promotion. In M. E. O'Connell, T. Boar, & K. E. Warner (Eds.), *Preventing mental, environmental, and behavioral disorders.* Washington, DC: National Academic Press.

O'Connor, M. J., Frankel, F., Paley, B., Schonfeld, A. M., Carpenter, E., Laugeson, E. A., et al. (2007). A controlled social skills training for children with fetal alcohol spectrum disorders. *Journal of Consulting and Clinical Psychology, 74,* 639–648. http://dx.doi.org/10.1037/0022-006X.74.4.639

O'Dea, J. A. (2005). Prevention of child obesity: "First, do no harm." *Health Education Research, 20,* 259–265. http://dx.doi.org/10.1093/her/cyg116

Ohl, M., Mitchell, K., Cassidy, T., & Fox, P. (2008). The Pyramid Club primary school-based intervention: Evaluating the impact on children's social–emotional health. *Child and Adolescent Mental Health, 13,* 115–121. http://dx.doi.org/10.1111/j.1475-3588.2007.00476.x

Olson, L. (2011). Development and implementation of groups to foster social participation and mental health. In S. Bazyk (Ed.), *Mental health promotion, prevention, and intervention with children and youth: A guiding framework for occupational therapy* (pp. 95–115). Bethesda, MD: AOTA Press.

OSEP Technical Assistance Center on Positive Behavioral Interventions and Supports. (2010). *Positive behavioral interventions and supports.* Retrieved June 15, 2012, from http://www.pbis.org/main.htm

Owens, G., Granader, Y., Humphrey, A., & Baron-Cohen, S. (2008). LEGO® therapy and the social use of language programme: An evaluation of two social skills interventions for children with high functioning autism and Asperger syndrome. *Journal of Autism and Developmental Disorders, 38,* 1944–1957. http://dx.doi.org/10.1007/s10803-008-0590-6

Ozonoff, S., & Miller, J. N. (1995). Teaching theory of mind: A new approach to social skills training for individuals with autism. *Journal of Autism and Developmental Disorders, 25,* 415–433. http://dx.doi.org/10.1007/BF02179376

Passmore, A. (1998). Does leisure have an association with creating cultural patterns of work? *Journal of Occupational Science, 5,* 161–165. http://dx.doi.org/10.1080/14427591.1998.9686445

Patient Protection and Affordable Care Act of 2010, Pub. L. 111–148, 124 Stat. 119.

Petrenchik, T. M., King, G. A., & Batorowicz, B. (2011). Children and youth with disabilities: Enhancing mental health through positive experiences of doing and belonging. In S. Bazyk (Ed.), *Mental health promotion, prevention, and intervention with children and youth: A guiding framework for occupational therapy* (pp. 189–205). Bethesda, MD: AOTA Press.

Pinto-Foltz, M., Logsdon, C., & Myers, J. A. (2011). Feasibility, acceptability, and initial efficacy of a knowledge-contact program to reduce mental illness stigma and improve mental health literacy in adolescents. *Social Science and Medicine, 72,* 2011–2019. http://dx.doi.org/10.1016/j.socscimed.2011.04.006

Poulsen, A. (2011). Children with attention deficit hyperactivity disorder, developmental coordination disorder, and learning disabilities. In S. Bazyk (Ed.), *Mental health promotion, prevention, and intervention with children and youth: A guiding framework for occupational therapy* (pp. 231–265). Bethesda, MD: AOTA Press.

Poulsen, A., Rodger, S., & Ziviani, J. (2006). Understanding children's motivation from a self-determination theoretical perspective: Implications for practice. *Australian Occupational Therapy Journal, 6,* 78–86. http://dx.doi.org/10.1080/08856250802387398

Powell, L., Gilchrist, M., & Stapley, J. (2008). A journey of self-discovery: An intervention involving massage, yoga, and relaxation for children with emotional and behavioural difficulties attending primary schools. *European Journal of Special Needs Education, 23,* 403–412. http://dx.doi.org/10.1080/08856250802387398

President's New Freedom Commission on Mental Health. (2003). *Achieving the promise: Transforming mental health care in America.* Retrieved June 15, 2012, from http://www.mentalhealthcommission.gov

Puhl, R. M., & Later, J. D. (2007). Stigma, obesity, and health of the nation's children. *Psychological Bulletin, 133,* 557–580. http://dx.doi.org/1037/0033-2909.133.4.557

Rehabilitation Act of 1973, § 504 (amended, 29 U.S.C. §794).

Rickel, A. U., Eshelman, A. K., & Loigman, G. A. (1983). Social problem solving training: A follow-up study of cognitive and behavioral effects. *Journal of Abnormal Child Psychology, 11,* 15–28. http://dx.doi.org/10.1007/BF00912174

Rimmer, J. H., Rowland, J. L., & Yamaki, K. (2007). Obesity and secondary conditions in adolescents with disabilities: Addressing the needs of an underserved population. *Journal of Adolescent Health, 41,* 224–229. http://dx.doi.org/10.1016/j.jadohealth.2007.05.005

Robertson, S. B., & Weistmer, S. E. (1997). The influence of peer models on the play scripts of children with specific language impairment. *Journal of Speech, Language, and Hearing Research, 40,* 49–61.

Rogers, J. C., & Holm, M. B. (2009). The occupational therapy process. In E. B. Crepeau, E. S. Cohn, & B. A. B. Schell (Eds.), *Willard and*

Spackman's occupational therapy (11th ed., pp. 479–518). Philadelphia: Lippincott Williams & Wilkins.

Sachs, J. J., & Miller, S. R. (2001). The impact of a wilderness experience on the social interaction and social expectations of behaviorally disordered adolescents. *Behavioral Disorders, 17,* 89–98.

Sackett, D. L., Rosenberg, W. M., Muir Gray, J. A., Haynes, R. B., & Richardson, W. S. (1996). Evidence-based medicine: What it is and what it isn't. *British Medical Journal, 312,* 71–72. http://dx.doi.org/10.1136/bmj.312.7023.71

Safran, S. P., & Oswald, K. (2003). Positive behavior supports: Can schools reshape disciplinary practices? *Exceptional Children, 69,* 361–373.

Santomier, J., & Kopczuk, W. (1981). Facilitation of interactions between retarded and nonretarded students in a physical education setting. *Education and Training of the Mentally Retarded, 16*(1), 20–23.

Santor, D. A., Poulin, C., Leblanc, J., & Kususmakar, V. (2007). Adolescent help seeking behavior on the Internet: Opportunities for health promotion and early identification of difficulties. *Journal of the American Academy of Child and Adolescent Psychiatry, 46,* 50–59. http://dx.doi.org/10.1097/01.chi.0000242247.45919.ee

Schery, T. K., & O'Connor, L. C. (1992). The effectiveness of school-based computer language intervention with severely handicapped children. *Language, Speech, and Hearing Services in Schools, 23,* 43–47.

Schilling, E. A., Aseltine, R. H., Glanovsky, J. L., James, A., & Jacobs, D. (2009). Adolescent alcohol use, suicidal ideation, and suicide attempts. *Journal of Adolescent Health, 44,* 335–341. http://dx.doi.org/10.1016/j.jadohealth.2008.08.006

Schleien, S. J., Mustonen, T., & Rynders, J. E. (1995). Participation of children with autism and nondisabled peers in a cooperatively structured community art program. *Journal of Autism and Developmental Disorders, 25,* 397–413. http://dx.doi.org/10.1007/BF02179375

Schleien, S. J., Rynders, J. E., Mustonen, T., & Fox, A. (1990). Effects of social play activities on the play behavior of children with autism. *Journal of Leisure Research, 22,* 317–328.

Schwartz, C., Garland, O., Waddell, C., & Harrison, E. (2006). *Mental health and developmental disabilities in children.* Vancouver: British Columbia Ministry of Children and Family Development, Children's Health Policy Centre.

Schwartzberg, S. L. (2003). Group process. In E. B. Crepeau, E. S. Cohn, & B. A. Boyt Schell (Eds.), *Willard and Spackman's occupational therapy* (10th ed., pp. 171–184). Philadelphia: Lippincott Williams & Wilkins.

Sebian, J., Mettrick, J., Weiss, C., Stephan, S., Lever, N., & Weist, M. (2007). *Education and system-of-care approaches: Solutions for educators and school mental health professionals.* Baltimore: Center for School Mental Health Analysis and Action, Department of Psychiatry, University of Maryland School of Medicine.

Seligman, M. E. P. (2002). *Authentic happiness.* New York: Free Press.

Seligman, M. E. P., & Csikszentmihalyi, M. (2000). Positive psychology: An introduction. *American Psychologist, 55,* 5–14.

Serna, L., Nielsen, E., Lambros, K., & Forness, S. (2000). Primary prevention with children at risk for emotional or behavioral disorders: Data on a universal intervention for Head Start classrooms. *Behavioral Disorders, 26,* 70–84.

Shechtman, Z. (2000). An innovative intervention for treatment of child and adolescent aggression: An outcome study. *Psychology in the Schools, 37,* 157–167. http://dx.doi.org/10.1002/(SICI)1520-6807(200003)37:2<157::AID-PITS7>3.0.CO:2-G

Shechtman, Z., & Ben-David, M. (1999). Group and individual treatment of childhood aggression: A comparison of outcomes and process. *Group Dynamics, 3*, 1–12. http://dx.doi.org/10.1037/1089-2699.3.4.263

Shure, M. B. (2001). *Raising a thinking preteen: The I Can Problem Solve program for eight-to-twelve-year-olds.* New York: Owl/Holt.

Smallfield, S., & Anderson, A. J. (2009). Using after-school programming to support health and wellness: A physical activity engagement program description. *Early Intervention Special Interest Section Quarterly, 16*(3), 1–4.

Sparling, J. W., Walker, D. F., & Singdahlsen, J. (1984). Play techniques with neurologically impaired preschoolers. *American Journal of Occupational Therapy, 38*, 603–612. http://dx.doi.org/10.5014/ajot.38.9.603

Spencer, K. C., Turkett, A., Vaughan, R., & Koenig, S. (2006). School-based practice patterns: A survey of occupational therapists in Colorado. *American Journal of Occupational Therapy, 60*, 81–90. http://dx.doi.org/10.5014/ajot.60.1.81

Stein, B. D., Jaycox, L. H., Kataoka, S. H., Wong, M., Tu, W., Elliott, M. N., et al. (2003). A mental health intervention for school children exposed to violence: A randomized controlled trial. *Journal of the American Medical Association, 290*, 603–611. http://dx.doi.org/10.1001/jama.290.5.603

Steinberg, L. (2004). Risk-taking in adolescence: What changes, and why? *Annals of the New York Academy of Sciences, 1021*, 51–58. http://dx.doi.org/10.1196/annals.1308.005

Steinberg, L. (2007). Risk taking in adolescence: New perspectives from brain and behavioral science. *Current Directions in Psychological Science, 16*, 55–59. http://dx.doi.org/10.1111/j.1467-8721.2007.00475.x

Stermac, L., & Josefowitz, N. (1985). A board game for teaching social skills in institutionalized adolescents. *Journal of Child Care, 2*, 31–37.

Stevahn, L., Johnson, D. W., Johnson, R. T., Oberle, K., & Wahl, L. (2000). Effects of conflict resolution training integrated into a kindergarten curriculum. *Child Development, 71*, 772–784. http://dx.doi.org/10.1111/1467-8624.00184

Stiffman, A. R., Stelk, W., Horwitz, S. M., Evans, M. E., Outlaw, F. H., & Atkins, M. (2010). A public health approach to children's mental health services: Possible solutions to current service inadequacies. *Administration and Policy in Mental Health, 37*, 120–124. http://dx.doi.org/10.1007/s10488-009-0259-2

Stiller, B., Ross, S., & Horner, R. (n.d.-a). *Bully prevention manual—Elementary school level.* Retrieved June 15, 2012, from http://www.pbis.org/common/pbisresources/publications/bullyprevention_ES.pdf

Stiller, B., Ross, S., & Horner, R. (n.d.-b). *Bully prevention manual—Middle school level.* Retrieved June 15, 2012, from http://www.pbis.org/common/pbisresources/publications/Bully-Prevention_PBS_MS.pdf

Substance Abuse and Mental Health Services Administration. (2012). *Caring for every child's mental health.* Retrieved June 15, 2012, from http://www.samhsa.gov/children/

Sugai, G., Horner, R. H., Dunlap, G., Hieneman, M., Lewis, T., Nelson, C. M., et al. (2000). Applying positive behavioral support and functional behavioral assessment in schools. *Journal of Positive Behavior Intervention, 2*, 1–25.

Sussman, J. E. (2009). The effect of music on peer awareness in preschool age children with developmental disabilities. *Journal of Music Therapy, 46*, 53–68.

Swearer, S. M., Espelage, D. L., Love, K. B., & Kingsbury, W. (2008). School-wide approaches to intervention for school aggression and bullying. In B. Doll & J. A. Cummings (Eds.), *Transforming school mental health services* (pp. 187–212). Thousand Oaks, CA: Corwin Press.

Tankersley, M., Kamps, D., Mancina, C., & Weidinger, D. (1996). Social interventions for Head Start children with behavioral risks: Implementation and outcomes. *Journal of Emotional and Behavioral Disorders, 4,* 171–181. http://dx.doi.org/10.1177/106342669600400304

Toblin, R. L., Paulozzi, L. J., Gilchrist, J., & Russell, P. J. (2008). Unintentional strangulation deaths from the "Choking Game" among youths aged 6–19 years: United States, 1995–2007. *Journal of Safety Research, 39,* 445–448. http://dx.doi.org/10.1016/j.jsr.2008.06.002

Tomb, M., & Hunter, L. (2004). Prevention of anxiety in children and adolescents in a school setting: The role of school-based practitioners. *Children and Schools, 26,* 87–101

Topolski, T. D., Patrick, D. L., Edwards, T. C., Huebner, C. E., Connell, F. A., & Mount, K. K. (2001). Quality of Life and health-risk behaviors among adolescents. *Journal of Adolescent Health, 29*(6), 426–435.

Townsend, S., Carey, P. D., Hollins, N. L., Helfrich, C., Blondis, M., Hoffman, A., et al. (1999). *The Occupational Therapy Psychosocial Assessment of Learning (OT PAL) Version 2.0.* Chicago: Model of Human Occupation Clearinghouse. Department of Occupational Therapy, University of Illinois.

Trombly, C. A. (1995). Occupation: Purposefulness and meaningfulness as therapeutic mechanisms. *American Journal of Occupational Therapy, 49,* 960–972.

Tse, J., Strulovitch, J., Tagalakis, V., Meng, L., & Fombonne, E. (2007). Social skills training for adolescents with Asperger syndrome and high-functioning autism. *Social Journal of Autism and Developmental Disorders, 37,* 1960–1968. http://dx.doi.org/10.1007/s10803-006-0343-3

Ttofi, M. M., & Farrington, D. P. (2009). What works in preventing bullying: Effective elements of anti-bullying programs. *Journal of Aggression,* *Conflict and Peace Research, 1,* 13–24. http://dx.doi.org/10.1108/17596599920090003

Tuttle, J., Campbell-Heider, N., & David, T. M. (2006). Positive adolescent life skills training for high-risk teens: Results of a group intervention study. *Journal of Pediatric Health Care, 20,* 184–191. http://dx.doi.org/10.1016/j.pedhc.2005.10.011

Tyndall-Lynd, A., Landreth, G., & Giordano, M. (2001). Intensive play therapy with child witnesses of domestic violence. *International Journal of Play Therapy, 10,* 53–83. http://dx.doi.org/10.1037/h0089443

Udwin, O. (1983). Imaginative play training as an intervention method with institutionalized preschool children. *British Journal of Educational Psychology, 53,* 32–39. http://dx.doi.org/10.1111/j.2044-8279.1983.tb02533.x

U.S. Department of Health and Human Services. (1999). *Mental health: A report of the Surgeon General.* Rockville, MD: Author.

VanderWaal, C. J., Powell, L. M., Terry-McElrath, Y. M., Bao, Y., & Flay, B. R. (2005). Community and school drug prevention strategy prevalence: Differential effects by setting and substance. *Journal of Primary Prevention, 26,* 299–320. http://dx.doi.org/10.1007/s10935-005-5390-6

Vaughn, S. R., & Ridley, C. A. (1983). A preschool interpersonal problem solving program: Does it affect behavior in the classroom? *Child Study Journal, 13,* 1–11.

Vogel, C. L. (2008). Classroom design for living and learning with autism. *Autism: Asperger's Digest Magazine.* Retrieved June 15, 2012, from http://www.autismdigest.com/Portals/0/docs/Classroom(2)-AADMay08.pdf

Vreeman, R. C., & Carroll, A. E. (2007). A systematic review of school-based interventions to prevent bullying. *Archives of Pediatric Adolescent*

Medicine, 161, 78–88. http://dx.doi.org/10.1001/archpedi.161.1.78

Waddell, C., Hua, J. M., Garland, O. M., Peters, R. D., & McEwan, K. (2007). Preventing mental disorders in children: A systematic review to inform policy-making. *Canadian Journal of Public Health, 98,* 166–173.

Wade, S. I., Carey, J., & Wolfe, C. R. (2006). An online family intervention to reduce parental distress following pediatric brain injury. *Journal of Consulting and Clinical Psychology, 74,* 445–454.

Wahler, R. G., & Meginnis, K. L. (1997). Strengthening child compliance through positive parenting practices: What works? *Journal of Clinical Child Psychology, 26,* 433–440. http://dx.doi.org/1207/s15374424jccp2604_12

Walker, H. M., Kavanagh, K., Stiller, B., Golly, A., Severson, H. H., & Feil, E. G. (1998). First step to success: An early intervention approach for preventing school antisocial behavior. *Journal of Emotional and Behavioral Disorders, 6,* 66–80. http://dx.doi.org/10.1177/106342669800600201

Walsh, R. T., Kosidoy, M., & Swanson, L. (1991). Promoting social–emotional development through creative drama for students with special needs. *Canadian Journal of Community Mental Health, 10,* 153–166.

Walsh-Bowers, R., & Basso, R. (1999). Improving early adolescents' peer relations through classroom creative drama: An integrated approach. *Social Work in Education, 21,* 23–32. http://dx.doi.org/10.1080/02165470120106997

Waters, E., de Silva-Sanigorski, A., Hall, B. J., Brown, T., Campbell, K. J., Gao, Y., et al. (2011). *Interventions for preventing obesity in children.* Cochrane Database of Systematic Reviews, Issue 12, Article No. CD001871. http://dx.doi.org/10.1002/14651858.CD001871.pub3

Waters, E., Salmon, L, & Wake, M. (2000). The parent-form Child Health Questionnaire in Australia: Comparison of reliability, validity, structure and norms. *Journal of Pediatric Psychology, 25*(6), 381–91.

Watling, R., Koenig, K. P., Davies, P. L., & Schaaf, R. C. (2011). *Occupational therapy practice guidelines for children and adolescents with challenges in sensory processing and sensory integration.* Bethesda, MD: AOTA Press.

Wehmeyer, M. L., & Bolding, N. (1999). Self-determination across living and working environments: A matched samples study of adults with mental retardation. *Mental Retardation, 37,* 353–363. http://dx.doi.org/10.1352/0047-6765(1999)037<0353:SALAWE>2.0.CO:2

Weist, M. D., & Paternite, C. E. (2006). Building an interconnected policy–training–practice–research agenda to advance school mental health. *Education and Treatment of Children, 29,* 173–196.

Wells, J., Barlow, J., & Stewart-Brown, S. (2003). A systematic review of universal approaches to mental health promotion in schools. *Health Education, 103,* 197–220. http://dx.doi.org/10.1108/09654280310485546

Wentzel, K., Baker, S., & Russell, S. (2009). Peer relationships and positive adjustment in school. In R. Gilman, E. S. Huebner, & M. J. Furlong (Eds.), *Handbook of positive psychology in schools* (pp. 229–244). New York: Routledge.

Wiener, J., & Harris, P. J. (1997). Evaluation of an individualized, context-based social skills training program for children with learning disabilities. *Learning Disabilities Research and Practice, 12,* 40–53.

Wilcock, A. A. (2006). *An occupational perspective of health* (2nd ed.). Thorofare, NJ: Slack.

Wilcock, A. A., & Townsend, E. A. (2008). Occupational justice. In E. B. Crepeau, E. S. Cohn, & B. B. Schell (Eds.), *Willard and Spackman's occupational therapy* (11th ed., pp. 192–199). Baltimore: Lippincott Williams & Wilkins.

Wilfley, D. E., Tibbs, T., L., Van Buren, D. J., Reach, K. P., Walker, M. S., & Epstein, L. H. (2007). Lifestyle interventions in the treatment of childhood overweight: A meta-analytic review of randomized controlled trials. *Health Psychology, 26,* 521–532. http://dx.doi.org/10.1037/0278-6133.26.5.521

Williams, M. S., & Shellenberger, S. (1996). *"How does your engine run?": A leader's guide to the Alert Program for self-regulation.* Albuquerque, NM: TherapyWorks.

Witt, W. P., Kasper, J. D., & Riley, A. W. (2003). Mental health services use among school-aged children with disabilities: The role of sociodemographics, functional limitations, family burdens, and care coordination. *Health Services Research, 38,* 1441–1466. http://dx.doi.org/10.1111/j.1475-6773.2003.00187.x

Wood, J., Drahota, A., Sze, K., Van Dyke, M., Decker, K., Fujii, C., et al. (2009). Effects of cognitive behavioral therapy on parent-reported autism symptoms in school-age children with high-functioning autism. *Journal of Autism and Developmental Disorders, 39,* 1608–1612. http://dx.doi.org/10.1007/s10803-009-0791-7

Woodard, W. (2009). Psychometric properties of the ASPeCT–DD: Measuring positive traits in persons with Developmental Disabilities. *Journal of Applied Research in Intellectual Disabilities, 22*(5), 433-444.

World Health Organization. (1986, November 21). *Ottawa charter for health promotion.* Retrieved June 15, 2012, from www.who.int/healthpromotion/conferenced/previous/ottawa/en/

World Health Organization. (2001). *International classification of functioning, disability and health.* Geneva: Author

World Health Organization. (2004). *Promoting mental health: Concepts, emerging evidence, practice: Summary report.* Geneva: Author

Wright, R., John, L., Ellenbogen, S., Offord, D. R., Duku, E. K., & Rowe, W. (2006). Effect of a structured arts program on the psychosocial functioning of youth from low-income communities: Findings from a Canadian longitudinal study. *Journal of Early Adolescence, 26,* 186–205. http://dx.doi.org/10.1177/0272431605285717

Young, R. L. (2007). The role of the occupational therapist in attention deficit hyperactivity disorder: A case study. *International Journal of Therapy and Rehabilitation, 14,* 454–459.

Ziviani, J., Poulsen, A., & Hansen, C. (2009). Movement skills proficiency and physical activity: A case for Engaging and Coaching for Health (EACH)–Child. *Australian Occupational Therapy Journal, 56,* 259–265. http://dx.doi.org/10.1111/j.1440-1630.2008.00758.x

Subject Index

Note: Page numbers in italics indicate figures, boxes, and tables.

Citation Index

Catalano, Hawkins, Berglund, Pollard, & Arthur (2002), 9, 21, 32

Catterall, Dumais, and Hampden-Thomson (2012), 70

Champagne (2008), 130

Charlebois, Normandeau, Vitaro, & Berneche (1999), 41, 47, 97

Christian & D'Auria (2006), 48, 97

Christner, Forrest, Morley, & Weinstein (2007), 52

Collaborative for Academic, Social, and Emotional Learning [CASEL] (2009), 132, 133

Conduct Problems Prevention Research Group (2002), 27, 41

Conduct Problems Prevention Research Group (2007), 97

Cook et al. (2008), 58, 98

Coren & Barlow (2001), 48, 117

Cowen (1991), 21

Csapo (1986), 39, 40, 98

Csikszentmihalyi (1993), 131

Davidson (2005), 13

Daykin et al. (2008), 29, 82

De, Small, & Baur (2008), 136

Dehghan, Akhtar-Danesh, & Merchant (2005), 135, 136, 138

DeMar (1997), 24, 27, 82

Demir, Zdemir, & Weitekamp (2007), 134

Demir & Weitekamp (2007), 134, 135

Diener (2000), 52

Dobson, McDougall, Busheikin, & Aldous (1995), 58, 117

Dolgin, Somer, Zaidel, and Zaizov (1997), 49, 98

Downing (2011), 38

Drysdale, Casey, & Porter-Armstrong (2008), 40, 48, 99

Dubow, Huesmann, & Eron (1987), 41, 47, 99

Duffy & Fuller (2000), 41, 49, 100

Duncan, Forness, & Harsough (1995), 32

Dunn (1999), 131

Dunn (2000), 44

Dunn (2007), 130

Dunn, Brown, & Youngstrom (2003), 16

Durlak, Weissberg, and Pachan (2010), 24, 27, 82

Durlak, Weissberg, Dymnicki, Taylor, & Schellinger (2011), 24, 26, 83

Dworkin (2003), 131

Dworkin, Larson, & Hansen (2003), 26

Dworkin et al. (2003), 132

Dwyer, Baur, Higgs, & Hardy (2009), 135

Ebbeck & Gibbons (1998), 29, 83

Eccles & Gootman (2002), 26, 39

Elias et al. (1997), 23

Emerson (2009), 136

Emmer & Stough (2001), 25

Epp (2008), 53, 55, 117

Eshelman & Loigman (2004), 47

Espelage & Swearer (2003), 132, 133

Fantuzzo et al. (1996), 49, 100

Felitti et al. (1998), 9

Forness (2003), 31, 32

Forness, Kavale, MacMillan, Asarnow, & Duncan (1996), 31

Fox (1999), 138

Frankel, Myatt, Cantwell, & Feinberg (1997), 40, 48, 100

Freeman et al. (2006), 25, 31, 34

Frolek Clark & Kingsley (2013), 1

Galantino, Galbavy, & Quinn (2008), 28

Galantino et al. (2008), 83

Gangl (1987), 58, 118

Gebert et al. (1998), 48, 101

Geldhof, Cardon, DeBourdeaudhuij, & De Clercq (2007), 28, 84

Gencoz (1997), 40, 43, 47, 49, 101

Ginsburg & Kingery (2007), 52

Girolametto (1988), 43, 48, 102

Gold, Wigram, & Elefant (2006), 59, 61, 118

Goleman (1995), 23

Gowen & Walker (2009), 52

Graham, Rodger, & Ziviani (2009), 38

Greenberg et al. (2003), 22

Summary

A three-tiered public health model has been presented to envision and guide occupational therapy's role in addressing the mental health needs of children and youth in school, community, and health care settings. Applying such a model emphasizes the need to reconceptualize services for children and youth to include promotion and prevention in addition to the remediation of problems.

Although the emphasis of occupational therapy will vary depending on context, all efforts share a common belief in the positive relationship between participation in a balance of meaningful occupations and health. Evidence to support occupation-based services at each tier has been presented, providing support for activity-based programs that emphasize the development of social skills, participation in play/leisure/recreation, health promotion, and stress reduction.